Competency Workbook to Accompany

LIPPINCOTT'S TEXTBOOK FOR CLINICAL MEDICAL ASSISTING

Diane Herschfelt, RN, BS, MAHB

Sharon Brill, RN, BSN, PHN

LIPPINCOTT WILLIAMS & WILKINS
A Wolters Kluwer Company
Philadelphia • Baltimore • New York • London
Buenos Aires • Hong Kong • Sydney • Tokyo

Ancillary Editor: Doris S. Wray
Project Editor: Nicole Walz
Senior Production Manager: Helen Ewan
Production Coordinator: Pat McCloskey
Design Coordinator: Doug Smock
Compositor: Pine Tree Composition, Inc.
Printer/Binder: Victor Graphics, Inc.

9 8 7 6 5 4 3 2 1

ISBN: 0-7817-1468-0

Preface

This study guide is designed specifically for use in conjunction with the text, **Lippincott's Textbook for Clinical Medical Assisting** by Julie Hosley, Shirley A. Jones, and Elizabeth Molle-Mathews. It is a structured way for students to practice *before* they perform procedures, prepare for competency exams and application practice!

COMPETENCY PRACTICE

This section contains various vocabulary assessment, practice, and application exercises.

First, we begin with various vocabulary assessment exercises to help students (at this level) use and understand terms within each chapter and to spell and define them correctly. Then, we follow with critical thinking and case study exercises with related questions. This is the point where students begin to ***apply*** principles and concepts taught in lecture and actually ***practice*** and demonstrate what they have learned. This generally consists of short answer and fill-in-the-blank questions. Each chapter concludes with some type of innovative learning activity that involves the use of illustrations contained in the text. Activities here include a variety of labeling, forms completion, dosage calculation and instrument identification exercises.

COMPETENCY EVALUATION

Now is the time to ***evaluate*** what the student has learned in accordance with the AAMA standards.

Procedure Checklists

- list performance objectives, equipment and supplies and include outcomes, conditions, and standards
- identify purpose and procedures by name
- list procedural steps exactly as they appear in the textbook

Charting Exercise

This is a way for the student to summarize everything learned, taught, and practicedand actually document on a patient's chart.

ANSWER KEY

Guidelines for responding to critical thinking questions included here may vary and are in the Instructor's Manual. If needed, please see your instructor for a copy.

APPENDIX—EXTERNSHIP ASSESSMENT RECORD

A summary of outcomes can be used so that a record of classroom performance and externship can be maintained. An instructor can initial each outcome once you have completed it in the classroom. Once performed in externship, your internship supervisor can initial it as well.

STUDENT SELF-STUDY DISK

Contains more than 300 multiple choice test item practice questions that help prepare you for testing. No other textbook of this kind has one!

We hope you enjoy this workbook.

Diane Herschfelt

Sharon Brill

Contents

1

Asepsis and Infection Control

COMPETENCY PRACTICE

Vocabulary Assessment

Vocabulary assessment exercises help students to correctly spell and understand terms presented in the chapter.

Matching

Match the term in Part 1 with the correct definition in Part 2.

PART 1

1. virulent
2. microorganisms
3. infection
4. asepsis
5. carrier
6. vector
7. transient flora
8. infection

PART 2

a. _____ person who is infected with a transmissible disease but who is asymptomatic

b. _____ disease-carrying insect

c. _____ do not normally reside in a particular area

d. _____ highly pathogenic

e. _____ invasion of pathogens into living tissue

f. _____ condition in which pathogens are absent

g. _____ microscopic living organisms

Spelling Applications

Correctly identify and spell the terms that are defined in the following statements.

1. The temperature scale on which 0 degrees is the freezing point and 100 degrees the boiling point of water at sea level is called ______________________ ______________________________________.
2. The acronym OSHA stands for __________________ ______________________________________.
3. Any departure from wellness is called ____________ ______________________________________.

4. The medical term meaning an object or area is free from infection, and is commonly referred to as clean technique, is ____________________.

5. Microorganisms in the body that are required for the normal functioning of the various systems are referred to as ____________________.

6. The medical term meaning an object or area free from all microorganisms and is commonly referred to as "sterile technique" is ____________________.

Critical Thinking

Critical thinking exercises help students apply principles and concepts presented in the chapter.

Answer these questions on a separate sheet of paper.

1. Choose a disease from Table 1-1 and create a patient education handout that focuses on preventing the spread of the disease.
2. Identify what type of asepsis would be required for the following procedures and justify your answers: catheterization, rectal temperature, excision of cyst, and injection.

Case Studies

1. Mrs. Garcia comes into your office with a towel around her hand. She explains that she has cut herself with a paring knife. The wound is no longer bleeding and will not require suturing. The physician asks you to clean and bandage the wound and to explain to the patient how to care for the wound at home so that it will not become infected. The patient asks you why you are putting on sterile gloves since she is clean and has no diseases. How will you educate this patient regarding your use of gloves? What directions will you give her regarding infection control methods that she can use at home in the care of her wound?

____

____

____

2. You are a medical assistant in a family practitioner's office. The doctor asks you to review with the staff the appropriate personal protective equipment (PPE). Identify the various types of PPE. Describe three situations that would require the use of PPE and why they must be used.

____

____

____

Basic Writing Activities

Fill-in-the-Blank

1. The ____________________ issues guidelines for isolation precautions for all patients.
2. Shaking hands, sexual contact, kissing, direct contact with blood or body fluids, or inhaling contaminated air droplets are examples of ____________________ transmission.
3. ____________________ is a special governmental regulatory body created to oversee worker safety.
4. The ____________________ virus may lead to cirrhosis of the liver or severe liver dysfunction with an increased risk for liver cancer.
5. A ____________________ detects the presence of antibodies if the immune system has responded to a vaccine.
6. A surgical scrub should be performed for ____________________ minutes.

Short Answer

1. Identify seven items of information listed on an MSDS.

____

____

____

2. List six natural body protective defense mechanisms.

____

____

____

3. List six conditions that favor the growth of pathogens.

____

____

____

4. Explain how hepatitis B is spread through the health care profession.

____

____

____

Innovative Activities

Labeling

Using Figure 1-1 the student is to identify and define each link.

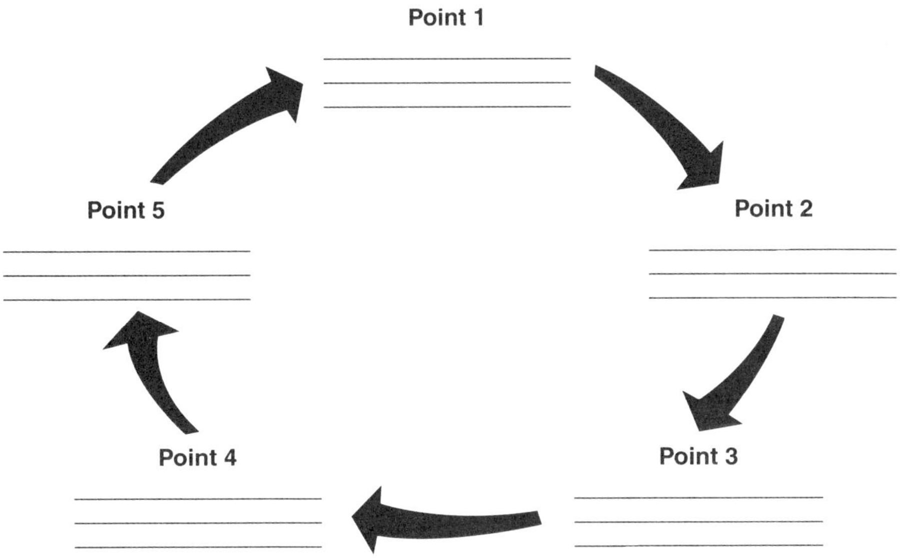

Figure 1-1

2

Medical History and Patient Interview

COMPETENCY PRACTICE

Vocabulary Assessment

Definitions

Write a term for each definition.

1. ______________________ objective indications of disease or bodily dysfunction
2. ______________________ traits or disorders that are transmitted from parent to offspring
3. ______________________ a disorder that tends to occur more often in a family than would be anticipated solely by chance
4. ______________________ description of the symptoms that lead a patient to seek physician's care
5. ______________________ medications that are available without a prescription
6. ______________________ subjective indications of disease or bodily changes as sensed by the patient
7. ______________________ process of gathering information about the patient and the presenting condition

Matching

Match the information in Part 1 with its location in the medical record in Part 2.

PART 1

1. patient takes OTC allergy pills
2. daughter had measles last year
3. mother died of breast cancer
4. father is living and well
5. brother is a dentist
6. patient smokes cigarettes
7. patient works in real estate

PART 2

a. _____ past history
b. _____ family history
c. _____ social history
d. _____ irrelevant

Critical Thinking

Answer these questions on a separate sheet of paper.

1. Mr. Green is a 35-year-old male who is scheduled for a physical examination with Dr. Allison. This is Mr. Greene's first visit to the office. The medical assistant is responsible for conducting the initial interview with Mr. Green to obtain pertinent information for the medical record. Identify and describe five interviewing techniques that the medical assistant can use when talking with Mr. Green.
2. The initial impression made by the medical assistant when greeting patients cannot be overemphasized. This impression sets the tone for any interview with the patient. Write an example of how a medical assistant can introduce herself or himself and explain the purpose of the interview.

Basic Writing Activities

Skill Drills

1. List the five different sections of the medical history and give examples of the type of information included in each.

____

____

____

2. List the four components of SOAP charting and give an example of each.

____

____

____

Innovative Activities

Form Completion

Interview a classmate and record appropriate data below.

____

____

____

____

____

____

____

____

____

____

____

____

COMPETENCY EVALUATION CHECKLIST

Procedure 2-1 Interviewing the Patient to Obtain a Medical History

NAME ______________________ **DATE/TIME** ______________

EVALUATED ______________________ **SCORE** ______________

Goal—To interview a patient to obtain a medical history.
Objectives/Conditions—When given a medical history form, pen, and any available previous information, the student will demonstrate interviewing skills to obtain needed information.
Outcome—A patient interview will be performed in accordance with the steps given in the text.

Equipment and Supplies

medical history form or questionnaire
previous medical information
pen

Steps	Y	N	Number of Attempts
1. Gather the supplies.	☐	☐	________
2. Review the medical history form.	☐	☐	________
3. Find a private and comfortable place.	☐	☐	________
4. Sit across from the patient at eye level and maintain frequent eye contact.	☐	☐	________
5. Introduce yourself and explain the purpose of the interview.	☐	☐	________
6. Using language the patient can understand, ask the appropriate questions and document the patient's responses. Be sure to determine the patient's chief complaint (CC) and present illness (PI).	☐	☐	________
7. Listen actively, stop writing from time to time, and look at the patient while he or she is speaking.	☐	☐	________
8. Regardless of the confidences shared by the patient, avoid projecting a judgmental attitude by your words or your actions.	☐	☐	________
9. If appropriate, explain to the patient what to expect during any examinations or procedures that may be scheduled for the day.	☐	☐	________
10. Thank the patient for cooperating during the interview and offer to answer any questions.	☐	☐	________

☐ Pass ☐ Fail

Comments

CHARTING EXERCISE

Mrs. Adams is a 33-year-old woman who is being seen in Dr. Apple's office for the first time. She complains of experiencing dizziness for the past 2 days. She takes no regular medication but does state that she fell and hit her head 1 week ago and questions whether the blow to the head could be causing her dizziness now. Mrs. Adams asks the medical assistant how Dr. Apple will assure the confidentiality of her medical record. What can the medical assistant tell Mrs. Adams about confidentiality? Document your interview with Mrs. Adams using a narrative format.

Document on the Patient's Chart:

- Date and time
- Notification of physician
- Patient complaints/concerns
- Patient education
- Your signature

Date/Time	Conditions/Lab Results Patient Communication

3

Anthropometric Measurements and Vital Signs

COMPETENCY PRACTICE

Vocabulary Assessment

Word Scramble

Unscramble the following words.

1. lnacrida nisgs

____

2. bifeler

____

3. ccley icradac

____

4. nptnhyeeisor

____

5. mrtitenet

____

6. sldoeait

____

Fill-in-the-Boxes

Fill-in the boxes with the correct term defined in each sentence.

1. pertaining to measurements of the human body

□□□□□□□□□□□□□

2. the contraction phase of the cardiac cycle

□□□□□□□

3. occurring at intervals

□□□□□□□□□□□□

4. measured against a standard

□□□□□□□□□□

5. sudden drop in blood pressure upon standing

□□□□□□□□□/

□□□□□□□□□□□

6. the original or initial measure by which other judgments are made

□□□□□□□□

Critical Thinking

1. Describe the effect of activity on blood pressure. Explain this effect on the procedure for obtaining a patient's blood pressure.

2. Explain how the size of the blood pressure can influence the measurement of a patient's blood pressure.

3. List and define eight different terms related to descriptions of respiratory rates.

Innovative Activities

Labeling

Please identify with an arrow the following temperatures: 37.8° C, 40° C, 99.2° F, and 102.1° F.

CENTIGRADE

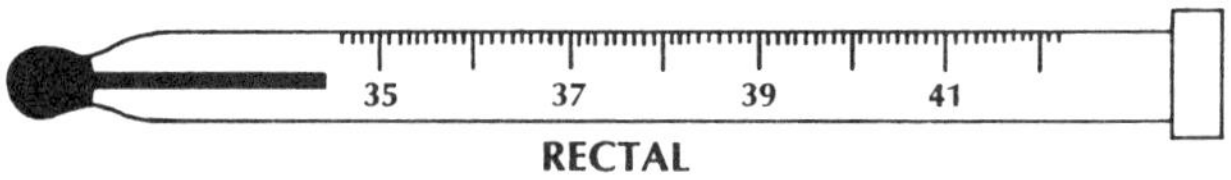

RECTAL

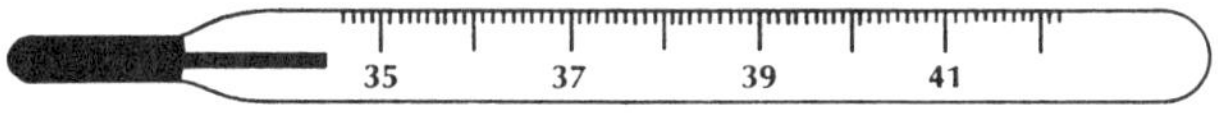

ORAL

FAHRENHEIT

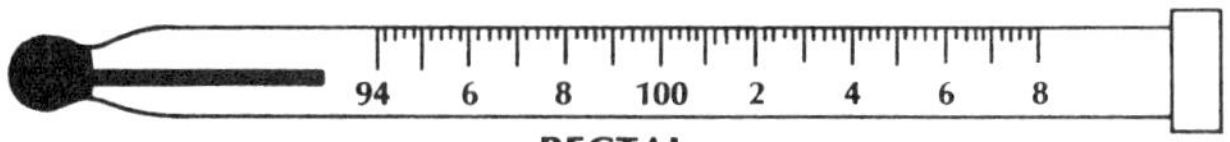

RECTAL

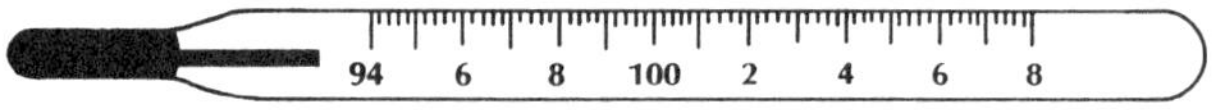

ORAL

Basic Writing Activities

Skill Drills

1. Identify and describe the four different types of thermometers.

2. List and describe the Korotkoff sounds and the five phases of blood pressure

COMPETENCY EVALUATION CHECKLIST

Procedure 3-1 Measuring Weight

NAME ______________________ **DATE/TIME** ______________

EVALUATED ______________________ **SCORE** ______________

Goal—To measure weight.
Objectives/Conditions—When using a calibrated scale the student will measure weight.
Outcome—The student will measure weight in accordance with the steps presented in the text.

Equipment and Supplies

calibrated scale
paper towel

Steps	Y	N	Number of Attempts
1. Wash your hands.	☐	☐	________
2. Ensure the scale is properly calibrated by observing that the balance beam hangs freely at midpoint when the counter weights are resting at zero.	☐	☐	________
3. Greet and identify the patient. Explain the procedure.	☐	☐	________
4. Escort the patient to the scale. Place a paper towel on the scale.	☐	☐	________
5. Make sure the scale is balanced at zero. (A balance beam scale should always be returned to zero after each use.)	☐	☐	________
6. Have the patient remove shoes, heavy coats or jackets, put down the purse, and step up onto the scale. *Note:* Certain circumstances require that the patient be weighed wearing only a gown. In this situation, ensure patient privacy by moving the scale to the examining room, where the gowned patient will be waiting.	☐	☐	________
7. Assist the patient onto the scale. Have the patient stand steady without touching anything; watch closely for a loss of balance.	☐	☐	________
8. Weigh the patient.	☐	☐	________

☐ Pass ☐ Fail

Comments

____

____

____

____

Procedure 3-2 Measuring Height

NAME ______________________ **DATE/TIME** ______________

EVALUATED ______________________ **SCORE** ______________

Goal—To measure height.
Objectives/Conditions—Using a scale with a ruler or standard marked or mounted on a wall, the student will measure height.
Outcome—The student will measure height in accordance with the steps presented in the text.

Equipment and Supplies

scale with ruler or standard marked or mounted on a wall

Steps	Y	N	Number of Attempts
1. Have the patient stand straight and erect on the scale, heels together, eyes straight ahead. (The patient may be measured on the scale facing the ruler, but a better measurement will be made with the patient's back to the ruler.) If the measurement is against a wall standard, the posture requirements are the same.	☐	☐	______
2. With the measuring bar perpendicular to the ruler, slowly lower it until it firmly touches the patient's head. Press lightly if the hair is full and high.	☐	☐	______
3. Read the measurement at the point of movement on the ruler. If the measurements are in inches (with smaller marks for 1/4, 1/2, and 3/4), convert the inches to feet and inches. (Example: If the point of movement reads 65 plus two smaller lines, read it as 65 1/2. Remember that 12 inches equal 1 foot; therefore, the patient is 5 feet 5 1/2 inches tall.)	☐	☐	______
4. At the completion of the procedure, assist the patient from the scale.	☐	☐	______
5. Return the balance bar on the scale to zero and return the measuring bar to a safe position for the next procedure.	☐	☐	______

☐ Pass ☐ Fail

Comments

____

____

____

____

Procedure 3-3 Measuring Oral Temperature Using a Glass Mercury Thermometer

NAME ______________________ **DATE/TIME** ______________

EVALUATED ______________________ **SCORE** ______________

Goal—To measure oral temperature using a glass mercury thermometer.
Objectives/Conditions—Using a glass mercury thermometer, the student will obtain an oral temperature.
Outcome—The student will measure oral temperature in accordance with the steps presented in the text.

Equipment and Supplies

glass mercury thermometer designed for oral use
tissue or cotton balls
disposable plastic sheath (if used)
gloves

Steps	Y	N	Number of Attempts
1. Wash your hands.	☐	☐	________
2. Assemble the equipment and supplies. Check the thermometer for chips or cracks.	☐	☐	________
3. Greet and identify the patient. Explain the procedure. Check for recent eating, drinking, gum chewing, or smoking.	☐	☐	________
4. Rinse and dry the thermometer if it has been stored in solution. Wipe it from bulb to stem.	☐	☐	________
5. Read the thermometer by holding it by the stem horizontal to your face and turning it slowly to see the mercury column.	☐	☐	________
6. If the mercury registers above 94°F, grasp the thermometer by the stem with the thumb and forefinger and snap the wrist quickly several times to shake the mercury down to about 94°F. Avoid hitting the thermometer against anything.	☐	☐	________
7. If using a clear plastic sheath, cover the thermometer now.	☐	☐	________
8. Put on gloves.	☐	☐	________
9. Place the thermometer under the tongue to either side of the frenulum.	☐	☐	________
10. Tell the patient to keep his or her mouth closed but caution against biting down on the glass column.	☐	☐	________
11. Leave the thermometer in place for 3–5 minutes. *Note:* The pulse and respirations may be taken at this time. (See Procedure 3-9, Procedure 3-10, and Procedure 3-11)	☐	☐	________
12. Remove the thermometer after the prescribed time. Remove and discard the sheath (if used) in an appropriate container or wipe the thermometer with a clean tissue or cotton ball from stem to bulb.	☐	☐	________

Steps (Continued)	Y	N	Number of Attempts
13. Hold the thermometer as before and note the reading.	☐	☐	________
14. Thank the patient and provide appropriate instructions.	☐	☐	________
15. Disinfect the thermometer according to the facility's policy. Remove gloves. Wash your hands.	☐	☐	________

☐ **Pass** ☐ **Fail**

Comments

____

____

____

____

Procedure 3-4 Measuring Rectal Temperature Using a Glass Mercury Thermometer

NAME ______________________ **DATE/TIME** ______________

EVALUATED ______________________ **SCORE** ______________

Goal—To measure rectal temperature using a glass mercury thermometer.
Objectives/Conditions—Using a glass mercury thermometer, the student will measure rectal temperature.
Outcome—The student will measure rectal temperature in accordance with the steps presented in the text.

Equipment and Supplies

glass mercury thermometer designed for rectal use
surgical lubricant
tissues
disposable plastic sheath (if used)
gloves

Steps	Y	N	Number of Attempts
1–7. Follow steps 1–7 as described in Procedure 3-3.	☐	☐	______
8. Spread lubricant onto a tissue, then from the tissue to the thermometer. Put on gloves.	☐	☐	______
9. Ensure privacy. Place the patient in a side-lying position facing toward the examination room door. Drape appropriately.	☐	☐	______
10. Expose only the buttock area. With the nondominant hand, lift the topmost buttock. Visualize the anus.	☐	☐	______
11. Touch the thermometer to the anus lightly. The anus will usually reflexively tighten against the intrusion. When the anus relaxes, insert the thermometer gently past the sphincter. Have the patient breathe deeply with the mouth opened.	☐	☐	______
12. **Insert the thermometer about 1 1/2 inches for an adult, 1 inch for a child, and 1/2 inch for an infant older than 2 months.** *Note:* Infants younger than 2 months should have temperatures taken by the tympanic or axillary method to avoid damage to the rectal canal.	☐	☐	______
13. Release the upper buttock and drape the sheet back over the patient. Hold the thermometer in place for 3 minutes.	☐	☐	______
14. At the end of 3 minutes, remove the thermometer. Offer the patient a tissue for cleaning or assist as needed. Remove the sheath by turning it inside out as it is pulled from the thermometer. Wipe the thermometer from stem to bulb. Discard sheath in appropriate container.	☐	☐	______

Steps (Continued)	Y	N	Number of Attempts
15. Note the reading. Remove and dispose of gloves. Wash your hands.	☐	☐	______
16. Thank the patient and provide appropriate instructions.	☐	☐	______
17. Disinfect thermometer according to the facility's policy. Wash your hands.	☐	☐	______

☐ **Pass** ☐ **Fail**

Comments

____

____

____

____

Procedure 3-5 Measuring Axillary Temperature Using a Glass Mercury Thermometer

NAME ______________________ **DATE/TIME** ______________

EVALUATED ______________________ ________ **SCORE** ________

Goal—To measure axillary temperature using a glass mercury thermometer.

Objectives/Conditions—Using a glass mercury thermometer, the student will measure an axillary temperature.

Outcome—The student will measure an axillary temperature in accordance with steps in the text.

Equipment and Supplies

glass mercury thermometer (either oral or rectal, according to facility's policy)
tissues
sheaths (if used)

Steps	Y	N	Number of Attempts
1–7. Follow steps 1–7 as directed in Procedure 3-3.	☐	☐	________
8. Expose the axillary area. Do not expose more of the patient's chest or upper body than is necessary to ensure the proper placement of the thermometer.	☐	☐	________
9. Dry the axilla with patting motions.	☐	☐	________
10. Place the bulb of the thermometer well into the axilla. Close the arm down over the axilla and cross the forearm over the chest. Drape the clothes or gown over the patient for privacy.	☐	☐	________
11. Leave the thermometer in place for 10 minutes. Stay with the patient.	☐	☐	________
12. Remove the thermometer after the prescribed time. Remove the sheath or clean from stem to bulb. Note the reading.	☐	☐	________
13. Thank the patient and provide appropriate instructions.	☐	☐	________
14. Disinfect the thermometer according to the facility's policy. Wash your hands.	☐	☐	________

☐ **Pass** ☐ **Fail**

Comments

____

____

____

____

Procedure 3-6 Measuring Temperature Using an Electronic Thermometer

NAME ______________________ **DATE/TIME** ______________

EVALUATED ______________________ ______________ **SCORE** ______________

Goal—To measure temperature using an electronic thermometer.

Objectives/Conditions—Using an electronic thermometer, the student will measure temperature.

Outcome—The student will measure a temperature using an electronic thermometer in accordance with steps in the text.

Equipment and Supplies

battery-powered unit with probes and covers
lubricant (for rectal temperature)
gloves

Steps	Y	N	Number of Attempts
1. Wash your hands.	☐	☐	______
2. Assemble the equipment and supplies.	☐	☐	______
3. Greet and identify the patient. Explain the procedure.	☐	☐	______
4. Choose the method most appropriate for the particular patient (eg, oral, rectal, axillary) and cover the probe to be used. Almost all units have one probe for oral and one for rectal. Covers are carried with the unit in a specially fitted box attached to the back of the unit. Put on gloves.	☐	☐	______
5. Place the thermometer as described for measuring an oral temperature (Procedure 3-3), rectal temperature (Procedure 3-4), or axillary temperature (Procedure 3-5).	☐	☐	______
6. If taking an oral temperature, help the patient hold the probe. If taking a rectal temperature, you must hold the probe.	☐	☐	______
7. Note that the electronic unit will emit a beep when the temperature shows no signs of rising beyond a certain point. This will usually be within 20–60 seconds.	☐	☐	______
8. Remove the probe. Note the reading; most will retain the reading until the probe is reinserted into the unit.	☐	☐	______
9. Discard the probe cover in a waste receptacle. If this was a rectal temperature, help the patient to clean away any remaining lubricant. Remove gloves. Wash your hands.	☐	☐	______

Steps (Continued)	Y	N	Number of Attempts
10. Thank the patient and provide appropriate instructions.	☐	☐	______
11. Return the unit to the charging base.	☐	☐	______

☐ **Pass** ☐ **Fail**

Comments

Procedure 3-7 Measuring Temperature Using a Tympanic Thermometer

NAME ______________________________ **DATE/TIME** ______________

EVALUATED ______________________________ **SCORE** ______________

Goal—To measure temperature using a tympanic thermometer.
Objectives/Conditions—Using a tympanic thermometer, the student will measure temperature.
Outcome—The student will measure a temperature using a tympanic thermometer in accordance with steps in the text.

Equipment and Supplies

tympanic thermometer
disposable probe covers

Steps	Y	N	Number of Attempts
1. Wash your hands.	☐	☐	______
2. Assemble the equipment and supplies.	☐	☐	______
3. Greet and identify the patient. Explain the procedure.	☐	☐	______
4. Remove the tympanic thermometer from the base and put the disposable cover on the probe.	☐	☐	______
5. Insert the probe, sealing the opening of the ear canal. Press the button to take the temperature, which will be displayed on the digital screen in about 2 seconds.	☐	☐	______
6. Remove the probe and note the reading. Discard the probe cover in a waste receptacle.	☐	☐	______
7. Thank the patient and provide appropriate instructions.	☐	☐	______
8. Return the unit to the base.	☐	☐	______

☐ **Pass** ☐ **Fail**

Comments

____

____

____

____

Procedure 3-8 Disinfecting a Glass Thermometer

NAME ______________________ **DATE/TIME** ______________

EVALUATED ______________________ **SCORE** ______________

Goal—To disinfect a glass thermometer.

Objectives/Conditions—When given gloves, soap, and soft tissue or cotton ball the student will disinfect a thermometer.

Outcome—The student will disinfect a thermometer in accordance with steps in the text.

Equipment and Supplies

thermometer to be disinfected
soft tissue or cotton ball
soap
gloves

Steps	Y	N	Number of Attempts
1. Put on gloves.	☐	☐	______
2. Wipe the thermometer with a soft tissue or cotton ball from stem to bulb with a rotating friction.	☐	☐	______
3. Rub the thermometer briskly with cool or tepid soapy water.	☐	☐	______
4. Rinse with cool water.	☐	☐	______
5. Dry well.	☐	☐	______
6. Place in the disinfectant soaking solution of choice, such as 70% alcohol.	☐	☐	______
7. After the prescribed period of time for the soaking solution of choice, remove the thermometer, rinse and store in a covered instrument tray padded with gauze to prevent chipping.	☐	☐	______

☐ Pass ☐ Fail

Comments

____

____

____

____

Procedure 3-9 Measuring Radial Pulse

NAME ______________________ DATE/TIME ______________

EVALUATED ______________________ SCORE ______________

Goal—To measure the radial pulse.
Objectives/Conditions—When given a watch with sweep second hand, the student will measure the radial pulse.
Outcome—The student will measure the radial pulse in accordance with steps in the text.

Equipment and Supplies

watch with sweep second hand

Steps	Y	N	Number of Attempts
1. Wash your hands.	☐	☐	______
2. Assemble the equipment.	☐	☐	______
3. Greet and identify the patient. Explain the procedure.	☐	☐	______
4. Place the patient in a seated or supine position with the arm relaxed and supported.	☐	☐	______
5. With the index, middle, and ring fingers of the dominant hand, use the fingertips to press firmly enough to feel the pulse, but gently enough not to obliterate it.	☐	☐	______
6. If the pulse is regular, count for 30 seconds and multiply by two. If this is a baseline pulse or if it is irregular, count for a full 60 seconds.	☐	☐	______

☐ Pass ☐ Fail

Comments

____

____

____

____

Procedure 3-10 Measuring the Apical Pulse

NAME ________________________ **DATE/TIME** ____________

EVALUATED ________________________ **SCORE** ____________

Goal—To measure the apical pulse.
Objectives/Conditions—When given a stethoscope and watch with a sweep second hand, the student will measure the apical pulse.
Outcome—The student will measure the apical pulse in accordance with steps in the text.

Equipment and Supplies

stethoscope
watch with sweep second hand

Steps	Y	N	Number of Attempts
1. Wash your hands.	☐	☐	______
2. Assemble the equipment. Ensure that the stethoscope has clean earpieces.	☐	☐	______
3. Greet and identify the patient. Explain the procedure.	☐	☐	______
4. Place the patient in a comfortable sitting or supine position. Remove the upper clothing or open sufficiently to allow access to the chest wall. Drape for privacy with a gown or sheet.	☐	☐	______
5. Locate the apex of the heart by palpating to the fifth intercostal space, between the fifth and sixth ribs. Move laterally to the left along the intercostal space to the nipple line or the midclavicular line.	☐	☐	______
6. Clean the stethoscope diaphragm with alcohol and warm it in the palm of your hand.	☐	☐	______
7. Insert the earpieces into the ear canals with the openings pointing slightly forward. A Doppler unit may also be used to broadcast the sound.	☐	☐	______
8. Position the stethoscope or Doppler unit until the sound is heard clearly. Listen for the S_1 and S_2 (sinus) sounds that will sound like "lubb, dubb." Together, they count as one beat.	☐	☐	______
9. Count for 1 full minute.	☐	☐	______

☐ **Pass** ☐ **Fail**

Comments

____

____

____

____

Procedure 3-11 Counting Respirations

NAME ______________________ DATE/TIME ______________

EVALUATED ______________________ SCORE ______________

Goal—To count respirations.
Objectives/Conditions—When given a stethoscope and watch with a sweep second hand, the student will count respirations.
Outcome—The student will count respiration in accordance with steps in the text.

Equipment and Supplies

watch with sweep second hand

Steps	Y	N	Number of Attempts
1. With patient already in position and sweep second hand in view, count a complete rise and fall of the chest as one respiration. *Note:* Some patients breathe at rest using the abdominal muscles more than the chest muscles. Observe carefully for the easiest area to assess for the most accurate reading.	☐	☐	______
2. If the pattern is regular, count respirations for 30 seconds and multiply by two, or count for 15 seconds and multiply by four. If the pattern is irregular, count respirations for a full minute.	☐	☐	______

☐ Pass ☐ Fail

Comments

____

____

____

____

Procedure 3-12 Measuring Blood Pressure

NAME ______________________ **DATE/TIME** ______________

EVALUATED ______________________ **SCORE** ______________

Goal—To measure blood pressure.
Objectives/Conditions—When given a sphygmomanometer, alcohol wipe, and stethoscope, the student will measure blood pressure.
Outcome—The student will measure blood pressure in accordance with steps in the text.

Equipment and Supplies

sphygmomanometer
alcohol wipe
stethoscope

Steps	Y	N	Number of Attempts
1. Wash your hands.	☐	☐	______
2. Assemble the equipment and supplies.	☐	☐	______
3. Identify the patient and explain the procedure. Ask the patient about recent smoking, caffeine, exercise, or emotional upset.	☐	☐	______
4. Position the patient. Have the patient's arm supported and slightly flexed with the palm upward. The upper arm should be level with the heart. The patient's legs should not be crossed, and the feet should be flat on the floor.	☐	☐	______
5. Expose the area. Remove the garment if the sleeve is too tight to raise above the area.	☐	☐	______
6. Center the deflated cuff over the brachial artery on the medial aspect of the upper arm. To assess the center of the cuff, fold the bladder in half; place the midpoint just above the brachial artery. The lower edge of the cuff should be 1–2 inches above the antecubital area.	☐	☐	______
7. Wrap the cuff smoothly. It should fit snugly against the arm without being too tight. (Cuffs vary. Some fasten with Velcro, some fasten with hooks, and others with long cloth tails.)	☐	☐	______
8. If using a mercury manometer, keep it vertical and at eye level. An aneroid dial must register with the needle at zero before beginning.	☐	☐	______
9. Palpate the brachial pulse with the fingertips of the nondominant hand in the antecubital area.	☐	☐	______
10. With the air pump in the dominant hand and valve between the thumb and forefinger, turn the screw clockwise (right to tighten). Do not tighten it to the point that it will be difficult to turn back.	☐	☐	______
11. With the fingers of the nondominant hand still at the pulse, inflate the cuff and note the point at which the brachial pulse is no longer felt. This number will be slightly below the first Korotkoff sound heard on auscultation.	☐	☐	______

Steps (Continued)	Y	N	Number of Attempts
12. Deflate the cuff by turning the knob counterclockwise (left to loosen). Wait at least 30 seconds before reinflating the cuff.	☐	☐	______
13. Clean the stethoscope chest piece with alcohol. Place the stethoscope earpieces in the ear canal with the openings pointing slightly forward. Stand or sit about 3 ft from the manometer, with the gauge at eye level. The stethoscope tubing should hang freely and should not rub against anything.	☐	☐	______
14. Place the bell or diaphragm against the brachial artery but do not press hard. Hold with the nondominant hand.	☐	☐	______
15. With the valve in the dominant hand, thumb and forefinger on the valve screw, turn the screw just tightly enough to inflate the cuff. Pump the valve to about 30 mmHg above the number felt on palpation.	☐	☐	______
16. With the thumb and forefinger remaining on the screw, slowly release the air at about 2–4 mmHg per second.	☐	☐	______
17. Listening carefully, note the point on the gauge at which the first clear tapping sound is heard. This is the first systolic sound or Korotkoff I.	☐	☐	______
18. Read at the top level of the meniscus (curved surface) of the mercury or at the number indicated by an arrow on the aneroid. Aneroid and mercury measurements are usually recorded as even numbers.	☐	☐	______

☐ **Pass** ☐ **Fail**

Comments

____

____

____

____

CHARTING EXERCISE

Mr. Lee, aged 62, has an 11:00 a.m. appointment on December 11, 1998. The appointment is for an annual physical examination. You take his vital signs and the results are: temperature 98.6°F, pulse 78, respirations 20, and blood pressure 130/86. Document this information using the following chart example.

Document on the Patient's Chart:

- Date and time
- Notification of physician
- Patient complaints/concerns
- Patient education
- Your signature

Date/Time	Conditions/Lab Results Patient Communication

4

Physical Examination

COMPETENCY PRACTICE

Vocabulary Assessment

Definitions

Define the following terms.

1. auscultation

2. bruit

3. fixative

4. inspection

5. mensuration

6. occult

7. PERRLA

8. range of motion

9. transillumination

Matching

Match the definition in Part 1 with the correct term in Part 2.

PART 1

1. inequality in size or shape
2. passive movement of joints
3. touching the body with fingers or hands

4. tapping or striking the body with hand or instrument to produce sound
5. simultaneous examination of the rectum and vagina by gloved examiner
6. equality in size and shape
7. to the side

PART 2

a. _____ symmetry
b. _____ peripheral
c. _____ palpation
d. _____ manipulation
e. _____ rectovaginal
f. _____ percussion
g. _____ asymmetry

Critical Thinking

1. Explain the difference between auscultation and palpation. In what order are these examination techniques performed during the physical examination? Why?

____

____

2. Explain the two main functions of the medical assistant during the physical examination.

____

____

Case Studies

1. Dr. Smith will be performing a genital examination on Mrs. Green. Mrs. Green had hip surgery 3 months previously and is apprehensive about the examination because she believes she will not be able to assume the lithotomy position for the examination. What would you say to Mrs. Green about the examination? What position could be used for the examination?

____

____

____

2. Miss Smith is scheduled for a complete physical examination with Dr. Brown. This is the her first visit to Dr. Brown's office. Miss Smith tells the medical assistant she is nervous about what the physician may find during the examination. How would you develop rapport with Miss Smith in preparation for the physical examination?

____

____

____

Basic Writing Activities

Skill Drills

1. List the three components of the physical examination.

____

____

____

2. List four responsibilities of the medical assistant at the completion of the physical examination.

____

____

____

3. List four basic instruments used during the physical examination and their function.

____

____

____

4. List the three types of scopes used to examine the rectum and sigmoid colon.

____

____

____

Fill-in-the-Blank

Fill-in the blank with the correct answer.

1. The Ayre spatula, or _______________, is a thin, flat, smooth piece of wood about 6 inches long. It is used during a pelvic examination.
2. A _______________ examination involves the use of the examiner's fingers.
3. A _______________ is a gel used to reduce friction and provide for easy insertion.
4. Normally the tympanic membrane is _______________ in color.
5. Ear wax is called _______________.

Innovative Activities

Labeling

Using Figures 4-1, 4-2, 4-3, 4-5, 4-6, 4-7, 4-8, and 4-9, identify each instrument and explain its use in the physical examination.

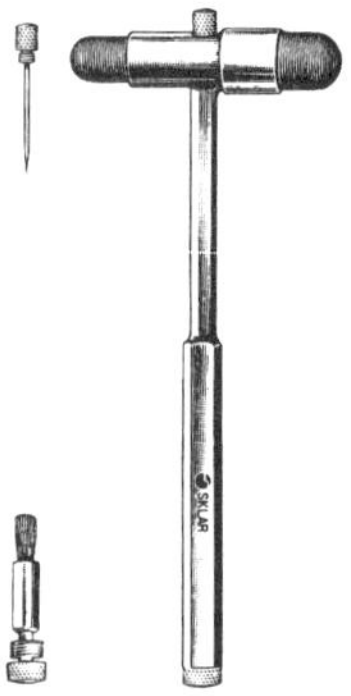
A

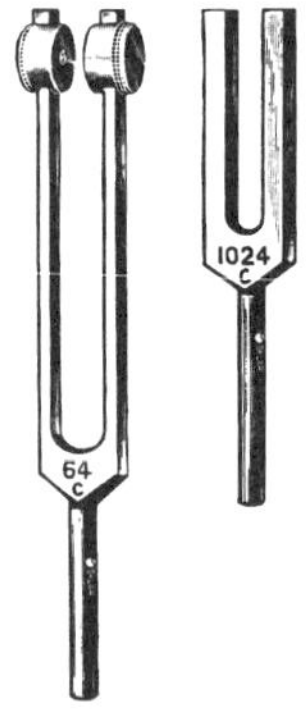
B

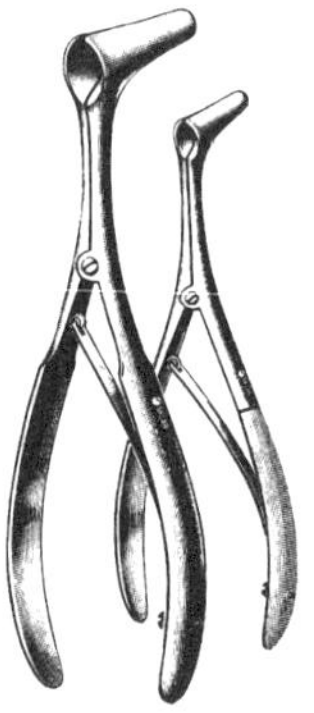
C

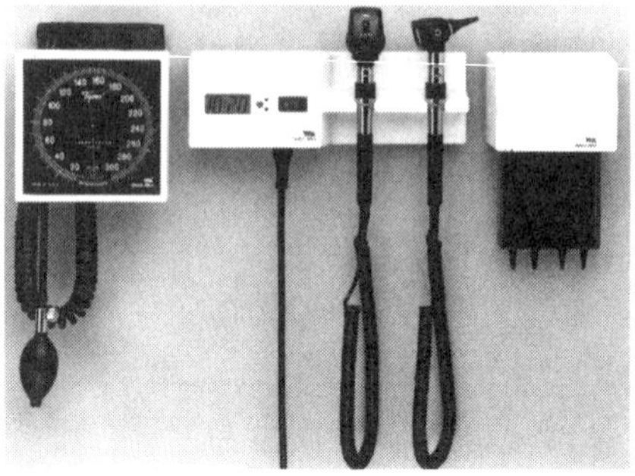
D

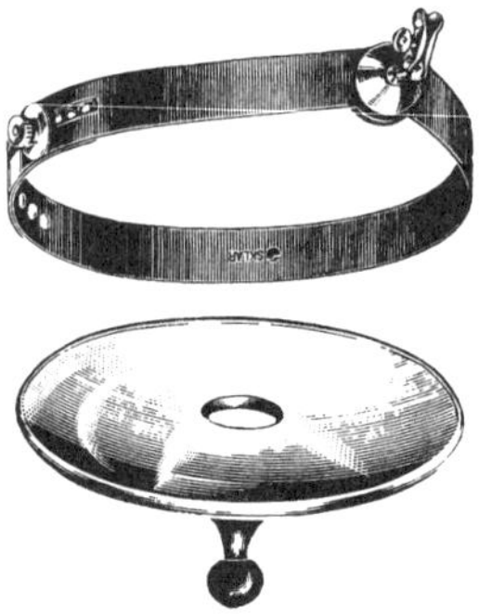
E

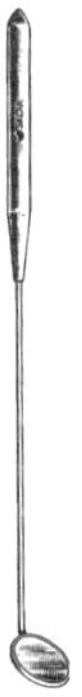
F

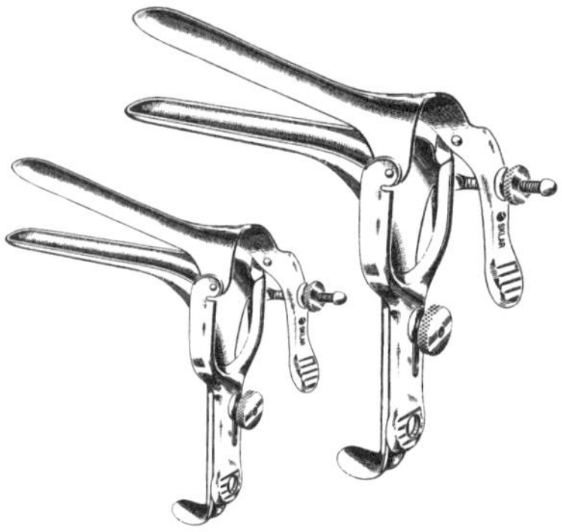
G

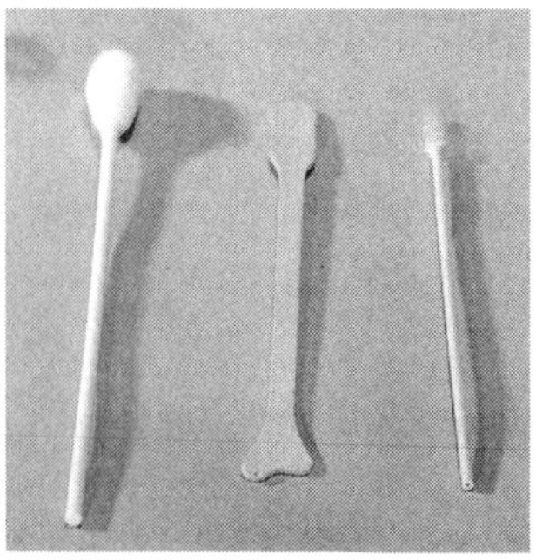
H

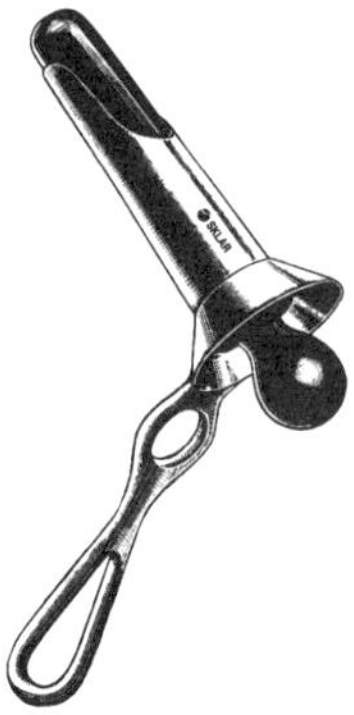
I

A. ____________________

B. ____________________

C. ____________________

D. ____________________

E. ____________________

F. ____________________

G. ____________________

H. ____________________

I. ____________________

Courtesy of Sklar Instruments, West Chester, PA.

COMPETENCY EVALUATION CHECKLIST

Procedure 4-1 Assisting With the Physical Examination

NAME ______________________ **DATE/TIME** ______________

EVALUATED ______________________ **SCORE** ______________

Goal—To assist with the physical examination.

Objectives/Conditions—When given equipment/supplies listed in the text, the student will assist with the physical examination.

Outcome—The student will assist with the physical examination in accordance with steps presented in the text.

Equipment and Supplies

stethoscope
ophthalmoscope
penlight
otoscope
tuning fork
nasal speculum
tongue blade
laryngeal mirror
percussion hammer
speculum
glass of water (optional)
substances for testing sense of smell (optional)
gloves
gauze squares
lubricant
vaginal specula/histobrush
slides, slide covers, and fixative
requisition slips as appropriate
tissues
specimen container
gown
drape
electrocardiograph

Steps	Y	N	Number of Attempts
1. Wash your hands.	☐	☐	________
2. Prepare the examining room.	☐	☐	________
3. Assemble the equipment.	☐	☐	________
4. Greet the patient by name and escort to the examining room.	☐	☐	________
5. Explain the procedures.	☐	☐	________
6. Obtain and record the medical history and chief complaint if that is your responsibility.	☐	☐	________
7. Take and record the patient's temperature, pulse, respirations, blood pressure, height, weight, and visual acuity. Draw blood if necessary.	☐	☐	________
8. Instruct the patient in obtaining a urine specimen and escort to the restroom.	☐	☐	________

Steps (Continued)	Y	N	Number of Attempts
9. See that the specimen is properly labeled and received in the laboratory.	☐	☐	______
10. Escort the patient back to the examining room. Instruct patient to disrobe completely and put on a gown opening down the back or front as directed by the physician. Leave the room unless the patient needs assistance.	☐	☐	______
11. Perform an electrocardiogram if ordered.	☐	☐	______
12. Assist the patient into a sitting position on the edge of the examination table. Cover the lap and legs with a drape sheet.	☐	☐	______
13. Place the patient's chart outside the examination room door, and notify the physician that the patient is ready.	☐	☐	______
14. Assist the physician during the examination by handing the instruments needed for examination of each body area and ensuring proper patient positioning.	☐	☐	______
15. Help the patient to return to a sitting position at the edge of the examining table.	☐	☐	______
16. Perform any follow-up procedures or treatments.	☐	☐	______
17. Leave the room while the patient dresses unless needed for assistance with clothing.	☐	☐	______
18. Return to the room to answer questions, reinforce instructions, and provide patient education.	☐	☐	______
19. Escort the patient to the front office.	☐	☐	______
20. Properly clean or dispose of all used equipment. Clean the room with disinfectant and prepare for the next patient.	☐	☐	______
21. Wash your hands.	☐	☐	______

☐ **Pass** ☐ **Fail**

Comments

____

____

____

____

CHARTING EXERCISE

Mrs. Jones is a 65-year-old woman scheduled for a physical examination with Dr. Ellis. Mrs. Jones is 5 feet 7 inches tall and weighs 135 pounds. Her BP is 110/60, and her pulse is 88. Dr. Ellis wants a specimen for urinalysis and cardiogram done before he examines Mrs. Jones. Mrs. Jones asks why these tests have been ordered before the examination. Using the above situation, document your interactions with the patient, including any patient teaching.

Document on the Patient's Chart:

- Date and time
- Notification of physician
- Patient complaints/concerns
- Patient education
- Your signature

Date/Time	Conditions/Lab Results Patient Communication

5

Instruments and Equipment

COMPETENCY PRACTICE

Vocabulary Assessment

Matching

Match the instrument description in Part 1 with the correct instrument in Part 2.

PART 1

1. slender jaws used for grasping blood vessels
2. spring handle, serrated, for grasping tissue for dissecting or suturing
3. sharp or blunt instrument composed of opposing cutting blades, for dissecting different tissue types
4. small surgical knife, straight handle and a sharp convex blade edge
5. plain or toothed, sharp or blunt, used to hold open layers of tissue
6. two tips, the bottom one is longer and is flattened, blunt, and angled in order to fit under dressings
7. long, thin, rounded and blunt tip, used to gauge the depth of an operative area

PART 2

a. _____ scalpel

b. _____ retractors

c. _____ bandage scissors

d. _____ hemostat

e. _____ probe

f. _____ thumb forceps

g. _____ scissors (straight or curved)

h. _____ needle holder

i. _____ towel clamps

Definitions

Define the following terms.

1. autoclave

____

____

____

2. disinfectant

____

____

____

3. disinfection

4. germicide

5. instrument

6. sanitizing

7. sterile field

8. sterilization

Critical Thinking

1. Explain the purpose of steam in the autoclave process of sterilization.

2. Why is it necessary to sanitize instruments if they are going to be sterilized?

Basic Writing Activities

Short Answer

1. What is the difference between disinfection and sterilization?

2. Why is it important to keep an up-to-date master list of all instruments and supplies, including all purchases and replacements?

Skill Drills

1. List five types of forceps.

2. List four properties of wrapping material necessary for proper sterilization and storage of sterile instruments.

3. List six types of information that load or sterilization records should contain.

4. List four different disinfection agents.

Innovative Activities

Labeling

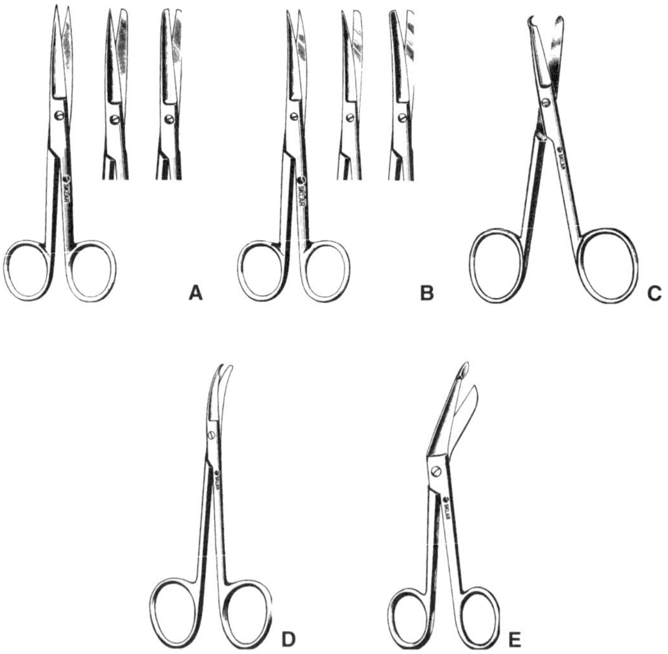

Identify each instrument.

A. ______________________________

B. ______________________________

C. ______________________________

D. ______________________________

E. ______________________________

Courtesy of Sklar Instruments, West Chester, PA.

COMPETENCY EVALUATION CHECKLIST

Procedure 5-1 Sanitizing Equipment for Sterilization or Disinfection

NAME ______________________ **DATE/TIME** ______________

EVALUATED ______________________ **SCORE** ______________

Goal—To sanitize equipment for sterilization or disinfection.

Objectives/Conditions—When given equipment and supplies listed in the text, the student will sanitize equipment for sterilization or disinfection.

Outcome—The student will sanitize equipment for sterilization or disinfection in accordance with steps in the text.

Equipment and Supplies

Equipment to be sanitized
Gloves
Impervious gown
Eye protection (goggles, face shield)
Soaking solution
Brushes or gauze
Basin

Steps	Y	N	Number of Attempts
1. Put on gloves, gown, and eye protection.	☐	☐	______
2. Take apart pieces that require assembly. If cleaning is not possible immediately, disassemble the pieces and soak the sections to avoid having them stick together.	☐	☐	______
3. Check for the operation and integrity of the equipment. If the equipment is defective, it should be repaired or discarded.	☐	☐	______
4. Rinse with cool water.	☐	☐	______
5. After the initial rinsing, force streams of soapy water through any tubular or grooved instruments to clean the inside and the outside.	☐	☐	______
6. After the cool rinse, use a hot soapy soak to dissolve fats or lubricants left on the surface. Use the soaking solution of choice for the facility.	☐	☐	______
7. Use friction with a soft brush or gauze to loosen transient microorganisms. Abrasive materials should not be used on delicate instruments and equipment. Brushes work well on grooves and joints. Open and close the jaws of scissors or forceps several times to ensure that all material has been removed.	☐	☐	______
8. Rinse well.	☐	☐	______

Steps (Continued)	Y	N	Number of Attempts
9. Dry well before autoclaving or soaking.	☐	☐	________
10. Be aware that any items used in the sanitation process (such as basins and brushes) are considered grossly contaminated and must be properly sanitized or discarded.	☐	☐	________

☐ **Pass** ☐ **Fail**

Comments

Procedure 5-2 Wrapping Equipment and Supplies for Sterilization

NAME ______________________ **DATE/TIME** ______________

EVALUATED ______________________ **SCORE** ______________

Goal—To wrap equipment for sterilization.

Objectives/Conditions—When given equipment and supplies listed in the text, the student will wrap equipment and supplies for sterilization.

Outcome—The student will wrap equipment and supplies in accordance with steps in the text.

Equipment and Supplies

Sanitized items
List of items to be included in pack, as needed
Sterilization wrap preferred by the facility, appropriate size for items
Sterilization indicator
Heat-sensitive sealing tape

Steps	Y	N	Number of Attempts
1. Open all hinged instruments.	☐	☐	________
2. Place a barrier cloth on the bottom of trays to be used as a surgical field.	☐	☐	________
3. If multiple items are to be wrapped together, place the larger, heavier items on the bottom.	☐	☐	________
4. If sharp pointed, hinged instruments are to be sterilized, place a cotton ball between the tips before wrapping.	☐	☐	________
5. Wrap the instruments.	☐	☐	________
6. Seal the items with sterilization indicator tape. Indicate on the tape the contents of the pack, the date of processing, and your initials.	☐	☐	________

☐ Pass ☐ Fail

Comments

____

____

____

____

Procedure 5-3 Operating an Autoclave

NAME ______________________ **DATE/TIME** ______________

EVALUATED ______________________ **SCORE** ______________

Goal—To operate an autoclave.
Objectives/Conditions—When given equipment and supplies listed in the text, the student will operate an autoclave.
Outcome—The student will operate an autoclave in accordance with steps in the text.

Equipment and Supplies

Sanitized, wrapped articles sealed with indicator tape (packs should each contain sterilization indicator)
Distilled water
Autoclave operating manual
Separately wrapped sterilization indicator

Steps	Y	N	Number of Attempts
1. Assemble the equipment. An indicator should be wrapped within each pack. An indicator may also be included and wrapped separately to check the efficiency of the process without disturbing the wrapped packages.	☐	☐	______
2. Check the water level and add more if needed, just to the fill line.	☐	☐	______
3. Load the autoclave:			
a. Place trays and packs on their sides, from 1 to 3 inches from each other and from the sides of the autoclave.	☐	☐	______
b. Put containers on their sides with the lids ajar.	☐	☐	______
c. In mixed loads, place hard objects on the bottom shelf and softer packs on the top racks.	☐	☐	______
d. Pack an indicator in the middle of the load.	☐	☐	______
4. Read the instructions that should be available near the machine.	☐	☐	______
5. When the load has cooled, remove the items. Wear thermal gloves to prevent burns.	☐	☐	______
6. Check the separately wrapped indicator for proper sterilization.	☐	☐	______
7. Store the items appropriately in a clean, dry, dust-free area. Site-prepared packs are considered sterile for 30 days.	☐	☐	______

Steps (Continued)	Y	N	Number of Attempts
8. Clean the autoclave by manufacturer's suggestions, which usually involve scrubbing with a mild detergent and a soft brush. Attention to the exhaust valve will prevent lint from occluding the outlet. Rinse the machine thoroughly and allow it to dry.	☐	☐	________

☐ **Pass** ☐ **Fail**

Comments

6

Assisting With Minor Office Surgery

COMPETENCY PRACTICE

Vocabulary Assessment

Matching

Match the term in Part 1 with the correct definition in Part 2.

PART 1

1. approximate
2. atraumatic
3. traumatic
4. coagulate
5. cautery

PART 2

a. _____ causing or relating to tissue damage

b. _____ a means, device, or agent that destroys or coagulates tissue

c. _____ to bring tissue surfaces together as closely as possible to their original positions

d. _____ without injury

e. _____ to change from a liquid to a solid or semi-solid mass

Definitions

Define each of the following terms.

1. bandage

____

____

____

2. dressing

____

____

____

3. preservative

____

____

____

4. ratchets

____

____

____

5. electrode

6. swaged needle

Critical Thinking

1. What precautions will you take when you are to shave and prepare a skin site prior to a minor surgical procedure?

2. Why might the physician choose to add epinephrine to local anesthetics?

Case Studies

1. Mr. Allen Johnson has a small laceration on the medial lateral aspect of his lower right leg, about 4 inches above the ankle, which he suffered when he fell off of his bicycle. The physician has sutured the wound. What type of dressing and bandage will you select, and how will you apply it?

2. Mr. Johnson tells you that he doesn't know what to expect regarding the healing of his leg wound, and he expresses concern about precautions he should take when he changes the dressing at home. How can you educate this patient to wound healing and what will you tell him to do in order to protect the wound during a dressing change?

CHARTING EXERCISE

Using the situation described in Case Study #2, please give an example of a chart note you might write following patient teaching.

Document on the Patient's Chart:

- Date and time
- Notification of physician
- Patient complaints/concerns
- Patient education
- Your signature

Date/Time	Conditions/Lab Results Patient Communication

Basic Writing Activities

Fill-in-the-Blanks

1. Steristrips are placed ________________ across the line of the wound.
2. Handles of transfer forceps are considered ________________.
3. If a package sterilized in the medical office becomes moist, it must be ________________ and ________________.
4. Before positioning the patient for a minor surgical procedure, have the patient ________________.
5. ________________ destroys tissue using controlled electric sparks.
6. Staple removal is a ________________ procedure.

Skill Drills

1. List the nine guidelines to follow during a sterile procedure.

____

____

____

2. List three common local anesthetics used in the medical office.

____

____

____

3. Describe the three ways in which the contents of peel-back packages may be added to the sterile field.

____

____

____

4. Bandages are used for many purposes. List five possible purposes.

____

____

____

Innovative Activities

Labeling

Identify each type of wound healing.

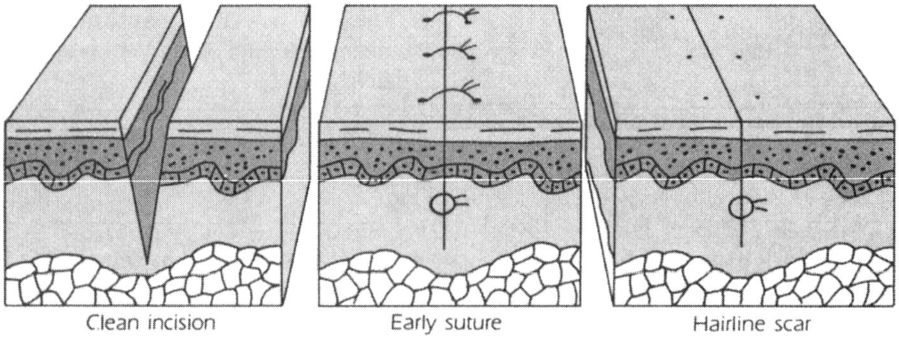

____

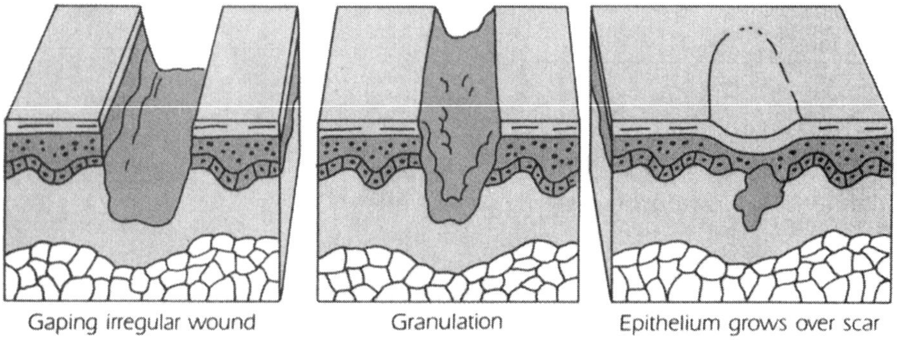

____

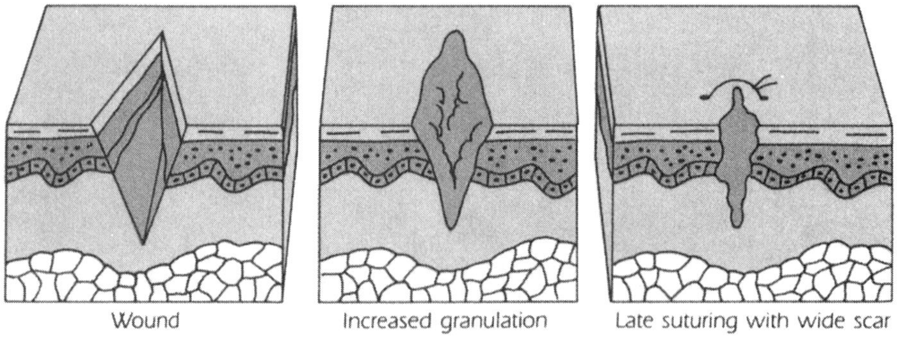

____

COMPETENCY EVALUATION CHECKLIST

Procedure 6-1 Opening Sterile Surgical Packs

NAME ______________________ **DATE/TIME** ______________

EVALUATED ______________________ **SCORE** ______________

Goal—To open a sterile surgical pack.

Objectives/Conditions—When given a sterile surgical pack, the student will demonstrate how to open the pack correctly.

Outcome—A sterile surgical pack is opened without contaminating the contents and in accordance with the steps presented in the text.

Equipment and Supplies

Surgical pack
Surgical stand

Steps	Y	N	Number of Attempts
1. Check the surgical procedure to be performed. Remove the appropriate tray or item(s) from the storage area.	☐	☐	______
2. Place the package, with the label facing up, on a clean, dry, flat surface, such as a Mayo or surgical stand.	☐	☐	______
3. Without tearing the wrapper, carefully remove the sealing tape. If the package is commercially prepared, carefully remove the outer protective wrapper.	☐	☐	______
4. Loosen the first flap of the folded wrapper. Open the first flap by pulling it up, out, and away; let it fall over the far side of the table.	☐	☐	______
5. Open the side flaps in a similar manner using the left hand for the left flap; right hand for right flap. Touch only the unsterile outer surface; do not touch the sterile inner surface.	☐	☐	______
6. Pull the remaining flap down and toward you by grasping the unsterile surface only. The unsterile surface of the wrapper is now against the surgical stand; the sterile inside surface of the wrapper forms the sterile field.	☐	☐	______
7. Repeat steps 4 through 6 for packages with a second or inside wrapper. This sterile inside wrapper also provides a sterile field on which to work. The field is now ready for additional supplies as needed or is ready for the procedure to begin.	☐	☐	______

☐ **Pass** ☐ **Fail**

Comments

____

____

____

____

Procedure 6-2 Using Sterile Transfer Forceps

NAME ________________________ **DATE/TIME** ____________

EVALUATED ________________________ **SCORE** ____________

Goal—To use sterile transfer forceps.

Objectives/Conditions—When given transfer forceps, forceps container, and items to be transferred, the student will correctly remove the transfer forceps from the container and transfer items from one area to another.

Outcome—Sterile transfer forceps are used without breaching sterile technique and in accordance with the steps presented in the text.

Equipment and Supplies

Forceps and container
Item(s) to be transferred

Steps	Y	N	Number of Attempts
1. Slowly lift the forceps straight up and out of the container without touching the inside above the level of the solution or the outside of the container.	☐	☐	____________
2. Hold the forceps with the tips down.	☐	☐	____________
3. Keep the forceps above waist level.	☐	☐	____________
4. Pick up the article to be transferred and drop it onto the sterile field so that the forceps will not come in contact with the sterile field.	☐	☐	____________

☐ **Pass** ☐ **Fail**

Comments

____

____

____

____

Procedure 6-3 Adding Sterile Solution to the Field

NAME ______________________ **DATE/TIME** ______________

EVALUATED ______________________ **SCORE** ______________

Goal—To add a sterile solution to the surgical field.
Objectives/Conditions—When given a sterile solution, the student will correctly add the solution to the surgical field.
Outcome—A sterile solution is added to the field without breaching sterile technique and in accordance with the steps presented in the text.

Equipment and Supplies

Container of sterile solution
Sterile setup

Steps	Y	N	Number of Attempts
1. As with any drug or medication, identify the correct solution by carefully READING THE LABEL.	☐	☐	______
2. Check for an expiration date on the label; do not use the solution if it is out of date, if the label cannot be read, or if the solution appears abnormal. *Note:* Sterile water and saline bottles must be dated when opened and must be discarded if not used within 48 hours.	☐	☐	______
3. If you are adding medications into the solution (eg, Xylocaine, a local anesthetic), show the medication label to the physician now.	☐	☐	______
4. With sterile transfer forceps, move any solution receptacles close to the edge of the sterile field but well within the 1-inch border.	☐	☐	______
5. Remove the cap or stopper. Hold the cap with the fingertips, with the cap opening facing downward, to prevent accidental contamination of the inside. If it is necessary to put the cap down, place it with the opened end facing up. If you are pouring the entire contents of the container onto the sterile field, you may discard the cap. Retain the bottle to keep track of amount added to the field and for charting purposes later. You can then discard it.	☐	☐	______
6. Grasp the container so that the label is facing the palm of the hand ("palm the label").	☐	☐	______
7. Pour a small amount of the solution into a separate container or waste receptacle.	☐	☐	______
8. Carefully and slowly pour the desired amount of solution into the sterile container from not less than 4 inches and not more than 6 inches above the container. Do not allow the bottle of solution to touch the sterile container or tray because this will cause contamination.	☐	☐	______
9. After pouring the desired amount of solution into the sterile container, recheck the label for contents and expiration date.	☐	☐	______

Steps (Continued)	Y	N	Number of Attempts
10. Replace the cap carefully to avoid touching the bottle rim with any unsterile surface of the cap.	☐	☐	______
11. Return the solution to its proper storage area and recheck the label again.	☐	☐	______

☐ **Pass** ☐ **Fail**

Comments

______

______

______

______

Procedure 6-4 Performing Hair Removal and Skin Preparation

NAME ______________________________ **DATE/TIME** ______________

EVALUATED ______________________________ **SCORE** ______________

Goal—To remove hair from the surgical area and to perform skin preparation.

Objectives/Conditions—When appropriate equipment is obtained, the student will correctly remove hair from a surgical area and complete skin preparation.

Outcome—Hair from a surgical area is removed and skin preparation is completed in accordance with the steps presented in the text.

Equipment and Supplies

Nonsterile gloves
Shave cream or lotion
New razor
Gauze or cotton balls and warm rinse water
Antiseptic
Sponge forceps

Steps	Y	N	Number of Attempts
1. Wash your hands.	☐	☐	______
2. Assemble the equipment.	☐	☐	______
3. Greet and identify the patient. Explain the procedure and answer any questions.	☐	☐	______
4. Put on gloves.	☐	☐	______
5. Prepare the patient's skin.	☐	☐	______
6. Apply antiseptic solution of the physician's choice to the skin surrounding the operative area using sterile gauze sponges, sterile cotton balls, or antiseptic wipes.	☐	☐	______
7. With dry sterile gauze sponges grasped in the sponge forceps, pat the area thoroughly dry. In some instances, the area may be allowed to air dry.	☐	☐	______
8. Instruct the patient not to touch or cover the prepared area.	☐	☐	______
9. Drape the prepared area for the procedure or cover it with sterile drapes if the procedure will be delayed for a short time. Longer delays may require reapplication of the antiseptic solution.	☐	☐	______

☐ Pass ☐ Fail

Comments

____
____
____
____

Procedure 6-5 Removing Sutures

NAME ______________________ **DATE/TIME** ______________

EVALUATED ______________________ **SCORE** ______________

Goal—To remove sutures from an operative site.

Objectives/Conditions—When appropriate equipment and supplies are obtained, the student will correctly demonstrate how to remove sutures.

Outcome—Sutures are removed using correct technique and in accordance with the steps presented in the text.

Equipment and Supplies

Thumb forceps
Antiseptic
Suture scissors
Gauze
Sterile gloves
Option: Sterile, disposable suture removal kits contain all needed supplies

Steps	Y	N	Number of Attempts
1. Wash your hands.	☐	☐	______
2. Assemble the equipment.	☐	☐	______
3. Greet and identify the patient. Explain the procedure and answer any questions.	☐	☐	______
4. If dressings have not been removed previously, do so (see Procedure 6-8). Properly dispose of dressings. *Note:* At this point in the procedure, the physician may be called to assess the healing process. The wound may need to be assessed both before and after exudate is removed. Then clean the wound area as directed.	☐	☐	______
5. Open the suture removal packet using surgical asepsis or set up a field for on-site sterile equipment. Put on sterile gloves.	☐	☐	______
6. Note that the knots will be tied in such a way that one tail of the knot will be very close to the surface of the skin while the other will be closer to the area of suture that is looped over the incision.	☐	☐	______
7. Remove the sutures.	☐	☐	______
8. Place the suture on a gauze sponge. Repeat the procedure for each suture.	☐	☐	______
9. Clean the site with an antiseptic solution, and if the physician has indicated, cover with a sterile dressing.	☐	☐	______
10. Properly care for or dispose of equipment and supplies. Clean the work area. Remove gloves and wash your hands.	☐	☐	______

☐ **Pass** ☐ **Fail**

Comments

____
____
____
____

Procedure 6-6 Removing Staples

NAME ______________________ **DATE/TIME** ______________

EVALUATED ______________________ **SCORE** ______________

Goal—To remove staples from an operative site.
Objectives/Conditions—When appropriate equipment and supplies are obtained, the student will correctly demonstrate how to remove staples.
Outcome—Staples are removed using correct technique and in accordance with the steps presented in the text.

Equipment and Supplies

Antiseptic solution or wipes
Sponge forceps
Sterile gloves
Gauze squares
Instrument for removing staples

Steps	Y	N	Number of Attempts
1. Wash your hands.	☐	☐	______
2. Assemble the equipment.	☐	☐	______
3. Greet and identify the patient. Explain the procedure and answer any questions.	☐	☐	______
4. If the dressing and bandages have not been removed, do so (Procedure 6-8). Dispose of dressings properly in a biohazard container. *Note:* At this point in the procedure, the physician may be called to assess the healing process. The wound may need to be assessed both before and after exudate is removed.	☐	☐	______
5. Clean the incision with antiseptic solution using the previously described method for wound care. Pat dry using dry sterile gauze sponges.	☐	☐	______
6. Put on sterile gloves.	☐	☐	______
7. Gently slide the end of the staple remover under each staple to be removed. Press the handles together to lift the ends of the staple out of the skin and remove the staple.	☐	☐	______
8. Place each staple on a gauze square as it is removed.	☐	☐	______
9. When all of the staples are removed, gently clean the incision as instructed for all procedures. Pat dry. Dress the site if required by the physician.	☐	☐	______
10. Properly care for or dispose of all equipment and supplies. Clean the work area. Remove gloves and wash your hands.	☐	☐	______

☐ **Pass** ☐ **Fail**

Comments

____

____

____

____

Procedure 6-7 Applying a Sterile Dressing

NAME ______________________________ **DATE/TIME** ______________

EVALUATED ______________________________ **SCORE** ______________

Goal—To apply a sterile dressing.

Objectives/Conditions—When appropriate equipment and supplies are obtained, the student will correctly demonstrate how to apply a sterile dressing.

Outcome—A sterile dressing is applied, using correct technique and in accordance with the steps presented in the text.

Equipment and Supplies

Sterile gloves
Dressings
Scissors
Appropriate bandages and tapes
Any medication to be applied to the dressing
Option: Disposable dressing change kits contain all needed supplies.

Steps	Y	N	Number of Attempts
1. Wash your hands.	☐	☐	______
2. Assemble equipment.	☐	☐	______
3. Greet and identify the patient. Ask about any tape allergies before deciding on the type of tape to use.	☐	☐	______
4. With the size of the dressing and bandage in mind, cut or tear lengths of tape to secure the bandage. Set the tape aside in a convenient location.	☐	☐	______
5. Explain the procedure and instruct the patient to remain still during the procedure and to avoid coughing, sneezing, or talking until the procedure is complete.	☐	☐	______
6. Open the dressing pack to create a sterile field. Observe the principles of surgical asepsis. Many packets are designed to be opened by the peel-apart method.	☐	☐	______
7. a. If sterile gloves are to be used for the procedure, open the appropriate size package of sterile gloves. Using sterile technique, put on the gloves. (See procedure for applying sterile gloves in Chapter 1, Asepsis and Infection Control.)	☐	☐	______
d. If using a sterile transfer forceps to apply the dressing (the "no-touch" method), use sterile technique to arrange the dressing on the wound site, and do not touch the dressing or the site with the hands.	☐	☐	______
8. Using the already opened sterile dressings and principles of sterile technique, apply to the wound the number of dressings needed to cover and protect the wound properly. Be sure to place sterile dressings carefully on the wound; do not drag them over the skin into position.	☐	☐	______

Steps (Continued)	Y	N	Number of Attempts
9. Apply the bandage so that it completely covers the sterile dressing and conforms to the patient's contours. The bandage should extend at least 1 inch beyond the border of the dressing.	☐	☐	______
10. Apply the previously cut lengths of tape over the bandage in a manner that secures both bandage and dressing. Apply tape sufficiently to secure the bandage, but avoid overuse of tape. When the wound is completely covered, you may remove your gloves, or you may prefer to keep them on during the taping. Discard them in the proper receptacle.	☐	☐	______
11. When the patient is required to change dressings at home, provide appropriate instructions. Dressings and bandages should be kept clean and dry and changed when wet or soiled. Otherwise, dressings should be changed as frequently as instructed by the physician. *Note:* The physician will describe to the patient the signs of infection, such as redness, swelling, pain, or undue warmth at the site; what to do regarding excess bleeding or drainage; and how to manage any drains that might be present.	☐	☐	______
12. Assist the patient from the examination table.	☐	☐	______
13. Properly care for or dispose of equipment and supplies. Disposable articles contaminated with blood or wound drainage require special disposal protocol. Clean the work area. (See Chapter 1, Asepsis and Infection Control.)	☐	☐	______
14. Return reusable supplies (unopened sterile gloves or dressings, bandages, tape) to their appropriate storage areas; all others should be discarded correctly.	☐	☐	______

☐ **Pass** ☐ **Fail**

Comments

____

____

____

____

Procedure 6-8 Changing an Existing Sterile Dressing

NAME ______________________ **DATE/TIME** ______________

EVALUATED ______________________ **SCORE** ______________

Goal—To change an existing sterile dressing.

Objectives/Conditions—When appropriate equipment and supplies are obtained, the student will correctly change an existing sterile dressing.

Outcome—An existing sterile dressing is changed, using correct technique and in accordance with the steps presented in the text.

Equipment and Supplies

Sterile dressings and sterile gloves (for applying the new dressing)
Unsterile gloves (for removing the old dressing and bandage)
Skin antiseptic solution with sterile gauze squares or sterile cotton balls or premedicated antiseptic wipes of the physician's choice
Sterile basin (to receive the solution and gauze or cotton)
Tape, torn to appropriate lengths and set aside as in Procedure 6-7
Approved biohazard containers for contaminated waste

Steps	Y	N	Number of Attempts
1. Wash your hands.	☐	☐	________
2. Assemble the equipment.	☐	☐	________
3. Greet and identify the patient. Explain the procedure and answer any questions.	☐	☐	________
4. Prepare a sterile field. If using a sterile container and solution, open the package containing the basin using sterile technique and use the inside of the wrapper as the sterile field for the basin. Peel apart the wrappers for the gauze or cotton balls and flip them into the basin or use sterile transfer forceps to place them in the basin.	☐	☐	________
5. Prepare antiseptic solution by first pouring off a small amount of the solution into a waste receptacle; then pour the solution from the stock bottle into the sterile container on the sterile field.	☐	☐	________
6. Instruct the patient not to talk, cough, sneeze, laugh, or move during the procedure.	☐	☐	________
7. Wearing clean gloves, carefully remove the tape from the bandage by pulling it toward the direction of the wound. Large bandages that encircle a limb may first be cut with bandage scissors on the side of the limb away from the wound. Remove the old bandage and dressing. *Note:* If the dressing is difficult to remove because of dried wound exudate or blood, soak it with sterile water or saline for a few minutes to loosen it. Gently pull the edges of the dressing toward the center. Never pull on a dressing that does not come off easily; the healing process will be disrupted. If this procedure does not loosen the dressing or causes undue discomfort to the patient, notify the physician immediately.	☐	☐	________

Steps (Continued)	**Y**	**N**	**Number of Attempts**
8. Discard the soiled dressing in a biohazard container. Do not pass it over the sterile field.	☐	☐	______
9. Inspect and observe the wound for degree of healing, amount and type of drainage, appearance of wound edges, and so on.	☐	☐	______
10. Observing medical asepsis, remove and discard gloves. *Note:* At this point, the physician should inspect the wound before exudate or drainage is removed. Decisions must be made regarding the healing process. If a culture is ordered, it must be taken before the wound is cleaned to ensure the most reliable test results.	☐	☐	______
11. Put on sterile gloves. Clean the area with the antiseptic solution of the physician's choice. Clean in a circular motion from the wound site outward. If a circular motion is not appropriate for this wound, use sweeps of the antiseptic-soaked gauze from the wound outward. Discard the wipe after each stroke. Never return the wipe to the antiseptic solution or to the skin after one sweep across the area.	☐	☐	______
12. Replace the dressing using the procedure for sterile dressing application (Procedure 6-7).	☐	☐	______

☐ **Pass** ☐ **Fail**

Comments

______

______

______

______

Procedure 6-9 Applying a Tubular Gauze Bandage

NAME ______________________ **DATE/TIME** ______________

EVALUATED ______________________ **SCORE** ______________

Goal—To apply a tubular gauze bandage.

Objectives/Conditions—When appropriate equipment and supplies are obtained, the student will correctly apply a tubular gauze bandage.

Outcome—A tubular gauze bandage is applied, using correct technique and in accordance with the steps presented in the text.

Equipment and Supplies

Tubular gauze
Applicator
Tape
Scissors

Steps	Y	N	Number of Attempts
1. Wash your hands.	☐	☐	______
2. Assemble the equipment.	☐	☐	______
3. Greet and identify the patient. Explain the procedure and answer any questions.	☐	☐	______
4. Choose the appropriate size tubular gauze applicator and gauze width. Manufacturers of tubular gauze supply charts with suggestions for the most appropriate size to use for various body parts.	☐	☐	______
5. Select and cut or tear adhesive tape in lengths to secure the gauze ends.	☐	☐	______
6. Place the gauze bandage on the applicator.	☐	☐	______
7. Place the applicator over the distal end of the affected part (finger, toe, leg) and begin to apply the gauze. Hold it in place as you move to step 8.	☐	☐	______
8. Slide the applicator containing the gauze up to the proximal end of the affected part. Holding the gauze at the proximal end of the affected part, pull the applicator and gauze toward the distal end.	☐	☐	______
9. Continue to hold the gauze in place. Pull the applicator 1 to 2 inches past the end of the affected part if the part is to be completely covered. In many instances, the gauze will not be required to extend beyond a limb and may cover only the area around the wound.	☐	☐	______
10. Turn the applicator one full turn to anchor the bandage.	☐	☐	______
11. Move the applicator toward the proximal part as before.	☐	☐	______
12. Move the applicator forward about 1 inch beyond the original starting point. Anchor the bandage again by turning it as before.	☐	☐	______

Steps (Continued)	Y	N	Number of Attempts
13. Repeat the procedure until the desired coverage is obtained. The final layer should end at the proximal part of the affected area. Any extra length of gauze not needed can be cut from the applicator. Remove the applicator.	☐	☐	______
14. Secure the bandage in place with adhesive tape or cut the gauze into two tails and tie them at the base of the tear. Tie the two tails around the closest proximal joint. Use adhesive tape sparingly to secure the end if not using a tie.	☐	☐	______
15. Properly care for or dispose of equipment and supplies. Clean the work area. Wash your hands.	☐	☐	______

☐ **Pass** ☐ **Fail**

Comments

____

____

____

____

Procedure 6-10 Assisting With Excisional Surgery

NAME ______________________ **DATE/TIME** ______________

EVALUATED ______________________ **SCORE** ______________

Goal—To assist the physician in an excisional surgery.

Objectives/Conditions—When assigned to assist a physician in an excisional surgery, the student will obtain appropriate equipment and supplies and demonstrate how to assist correctly in this type of surgery.

Outcome—The student assists with an excisional surgery, using correct technique and in accordance with the steps presented in the text.

Equipment and Supplies

At the side
Sterile gloves
Local anesthetic
Antiseptic wipes
Adhesive tape
Bandages
Specimen container with completed laboratory request

On the field
Basin for solutions
Gauze sponges and cotton balls
Antiseptic solution
Sterile drape
Dissecting scissors or iris scissors
Scalpel blade and handle of physician's choice
Mosquito forceps
Tissue forceps
Needle holder
Suture and needle of physician's choice

Steps	Y	N	Number of Attempts
1. Wash your hands.	☐	☐	________
2. Assemble the equipment.	☐	☐	________
3. Greet and identify the patient. Explain the procedure and answer any questions.	☐	☐	________
4. Step up a sterile field on a surgical stand with the at-the-side equipment close at hand. Cover the field with a sterile drape if necessary until the physician arrives.	☐	☐	________
5. Position the patient appropriately.	☐	☐	________
6. Put on sterile gloves or use transfer forceps for the aseptic process.	☐	☐	________
7. Cleanse the site with sterile antiseptic solution in the manner described for skin preparation (Procedure 6-4). *Note:* The physician may do this before gloving. Some physicians prefer that the site be cleaned and made ready by an assistant; others prefer doing it themselves after gloving and using the supplies on the field. In all instances, the physician's preference takes precedence over any outlined procedure.	☐	☐	________

Steps *(Continued)*	Y	N	Number of Attempts
8. The physician will perform the procedure; you may be asked to assist during the procedure. This usually involves adding supplies as needed, watching closely for opportunities to assist the physician and comforting the patient, or putting on sterile gloves and passing instruments to the physician from the field. *Note:* If the lesion is to be referred to pathology for analysis, you will be required to assist with the specimen container during the procedure.	☐	☐	__________
9. At the end of the procedure, dress the wound using the procedure for applying a sterile dressing (see Procedure 6-7).	☐	☐	__________
10. Assist the patient from the table and offer to help with clothing as needed.	☐	☐	__________
11. Clean the examining room in preparation for the next patient. Discard all disposables in appropriate biohazard containers. Return unused reusable items to their proper place. Wash your hands.	☐	☐	__________

☐ **Pass** ☐ **Fail**

Comments

Procedure 6-11 Assisting With Incision and Drainage (I&D)

NAME ______________________ **DATE/TIME** ______________

EVALUATED ______________________ **SCORE** ______________

Goal—To assist the physician in an incision and drainage procedure.

Objectives/Conditions—When assigned to assist a physician in an incision and drainage procedure, the student will obtain appropriate equipment and supplies and demonstrate how to assist correctly in this procedure.

Outcome—The student assists with an incision and drainage procedure, using correct technique and in accordance with the steps presented in the text.

Equipment and Supplies

At the side
Sterile gloves
Local anesthetic
Antiseptic wipes
Adhesive tape
Additional sterile dressings
Packing gauze
Bandages
(If the wound is to be cultured, a culture tube will also be included at the side.)

On the field
Basin
Sterile cotton balls or gauze
Antiseptic solution
Sterile drape
Syringes and needles for local anesthetic (unless the physician prefers that the sight be numbered before gloving)
Commercial I & D set or scalpel, dissecting scissors or operating scissors, hemostats, tissue forceps, 4 × 4 gauze sponges, probe (optional)

Steps	Y	N	Number of Attempts
1–4. Follow steps 1–4 of Procedure 6-10: Assisting With Excisional Surgery.	☐	☐	________
5. Position the patient appropriately.	☐	☐	________
6–8. Follow steps 6–8 of Procedure 6-10: Assisting With Excisional Surgery.	☐	☐	________
9. At the end of the procedure, dress the wound using the procedure for applying a sterile dressing (see Procedure 6-7).	☐	☐	________
10. Assist the patient from the table and offer to help with clothing as needed.	☐	☐	________

☐ **Pass** ☐ **Fail**

Comments

____

____

____

____

7

Pharmacology

COMPETENCY PRACTICE

Vocabulary Assessment

Matching

Match the definition in Part 1 with the correct term from Part 2.

PART 1

1. two drugs working together
2. one drug decreases the effect of another
3. one drug prolongs or multiplies the effect of another
4. study of how drugs act within the body
5. study of action of drugs within the body from administration to excretion
6. action that delivers the drug into the bloodstream
7. moves drugs from the bloodstream into tissues of the body
8. physical and chemical alterations that drug undergoes within the body
9. eliminates the waste products of drugs

PART 2

a. _____ pharmacodynamics
b. _____ absorption
c. _____ excretion
d. _____ distribution
e. _____ metabolism
f. _____ pharmacokinesis
g. _____ antagonism
h. _____ synergism
i. _____ potentiation

Word Scramble

Unscramble the following words to form a term used in the text.

1. udrg

____

2. tnpteooinita

____

3. msrenysgi

____

4. hraylocmapog

____

5. tgnanaosmi

____

6. coynicashrpmaadam

____

7. kocmrhpaaienssi

____

Critical Thinking

1. Explain two ways a medical assistant can educate a patient about taking medications.

____

____

____

2. Identify a drug that you have taken by its chemical name and describe two indications for its use. (Use a PDR as a source of information.)

____

____

____

Case Studies

1. On 4/19/99 Mrs. Jones calls the office and requests a refill of her diazepam prescription. You check Mrs. Smith's chart and find that the original Rx was written on 11/19/98 and has been refilled four times. Explain whether Mrs. Smith would be able to receive another refill of diazepam and why.

____

____

____

2. Mr. Jones is given a prescription for Tylenol with codeine for a sprained ankle. He states that he is concerned about becoming addicted to medications. What can you tell Mr. Jones about this drug and its potential to become habit forming?

____

____

____

CHARTING EXERCISE

On December 1, 1999 Mr. Alexander calls the office to request a refill on his prescription for Benadryl 50 mg #30. He takes one tablet four times a day, if necessary, for allergies. Dr. Smith approves the refill and asks you to document the refill in Mr. Alexander's chart. Write a narrative chart note documenting the refill of Mr. Alexander's medication.

Document on the Patient's Chart:

- Date and time
- Notification of physician
- Patient complaints/concerns
- Patient education
- Your signature

Date/Time	Conditions/Lab Results Patient Communication

Basic Writing Activities

Skill Drills

1. List five commonly noted physical allergic reactions.

____

____

____

2. List four sources of information on pharmacology.

____

____

____

3. Name the four regulations that historically have affected the manufacture, sale, and prescribing of medications.

____

____

____

4. Identify five factors that influence drug action.

____

____

____

Fill-in-the-Blanks

1. A drug manufacturer has exclusive right to produce a drug for ____________________ years.
2. The Pure Food and Drug Act was passed in ____________________ and amended in ____________________.
3. The first name given to any medication is its ____________________ name.
4. During research and development of a drug it is given its ____________________ name.
5. Drugs are classified according to their ____________________ and ____________________ on the body.

Innovative Activities

Labeling

Identify the four indicated parts of a prescription.

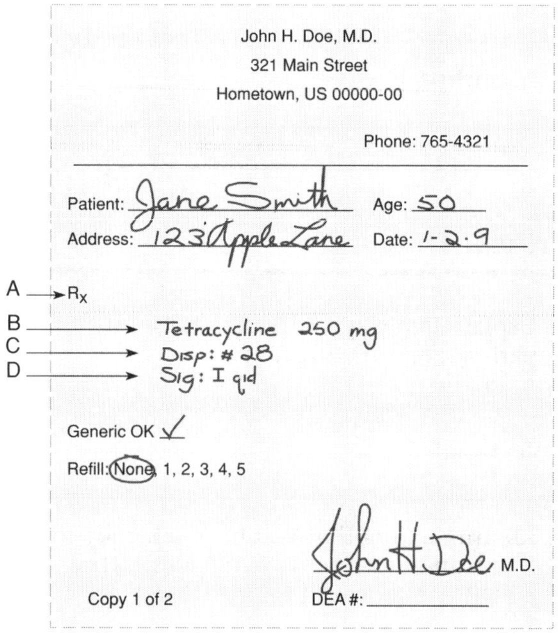

A. ____

B. ____

C. ____

D. ____

8

Preparing and Administering Medications

COMPETENCY PRACTICE

Vocabulary Assessment

Matching

Match the abbreviations in Part 1 with the correct definitions in Part 2.

PART 1	PART 2	
1. sig	a. _____	as desired
2. ung	b. _____	before meals
3. ad lib	c. _____	drop
4. stat	d. _____	nothing by mouth
5. pc	e. _____	whenever necessary
6. ac	f. _____	immediately
7. prn	g. _____	label
8. NPO	h. _____	ointment
9. gtt	i. _____	after meals
10. aa	j. _____	of each

Definitions

Define the following terms.

1. ampule

____

____

____

2. diluent

____

____

____

3. gauge

____

____

____

4. Mantoux

____

____

____

5. meniscus

____

____

____

6. nebulizer

____

____

____

7. vial

____

____

____

Critical Thinking

1. There are several formulas for pediatric dosage calculation. Describe the method considered to be the most accurate.

____

____

____

2. Oral and parenteral medications are absorbed into the body at different rates and in different ways. Describe a situation in which the parenteral route would be the one of choice.

____

____

____

Case Studies

1. Dr. Allen has ordered a tine test to be administered intradermally to Mr. Alexander as part of the patient's physical exam. Mr. Alexander states that he knows very little about this type of test, and as you give the tine test he asks you for information. How can you educate Mr. Alexander about the tine test? What patient instructions will you give?

____

____

____

2. Miss Jeffers is being seen today for complaints of "frequent indigestion and heartburn." At the end of the appointment Dr. Mathews asks you to give Tagamet 200 mg po to Miss Jeffers. You have in the medication cabinet a bottle of Tagamet 400 mg/tab. Using the ratio-proportion method, calculate the tablet dose required to deliver Tagamet 200 mg (show your calculations). You give the ordered medication.

____

____

____

CHARTING EXERCISE

Using the situation described in Case Study #2, please give an example of a chart note you might write following the administration of medication.

Document on the Patient's Chart:

- Date and time
- Notification of physician
- Patient complaints/concerns
- Patient education
- Your signature

Date/Time	Conditions/Lab Results Patient Communication

Basic Writing Activities

Skill Drills

1. List three types of injections and identify their angles.

____

____

____

2. Identify the steps necessary to correct a charting error in medication documentation.

____

____

____

3. List the "seven rights" of medication administration.

____

____

____

4. Explain what three items must be written on label when a powdered drug is reconstituted.

____

____

____

Fill-in-the-Blanks

1. A tuberculin syringe has a total capacity of ____________.
2. To change kilograms to pounds, multiply the kilograms by ____________.
3. An intramuscular injection requires a needle length of at least ____________.
4. Subcutaneous injections are usually given using a needle gauge and length of ____________.
5. Small glass medication containers that must be broken at the neck are ____________.
6. To change minims to cubic centimeters, divide the minims by ____________.

Innovative Activities

Labeling

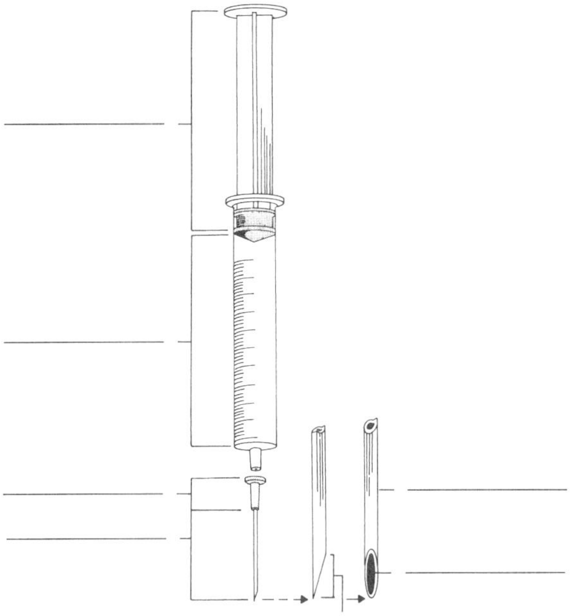

Identify the parts of a syringe and needle.

COMPETENCY EVALUATION CHECKLIST

Procedure 8-1 Administering Oral Medications

NAME ______________________ **DATE/TIME** ______________

EVALUATED ______________________ **SCORE** ______________

Goal—To administer an oral medication.

Objectives/Conditions—Upon receiving a physician order to give an oral medication, the student will obtain the appropriate supplies, other items, and the correct medication. The correct medication and dosage will be given orally to the right patient.

Outcome—An oral medication is correctly given in accordance with the steps presented in the text.

Equipment and Supplies

Medication
Medication tray
Disposable calibrated cup
Physician's instructions
Glass of water

Steps	Y	N	Number of Attempts
1. Wash your hands.	☐	☐	______
2. Assemble the equipment and supplies.	☐	☐	______
3. Select the medication. Compare the label to the physician's instructions. Check the expiration date. Check the label three times: when taking it from the shelf, while pouring, and when returning to the shelf.	☐	☐	______
4. Calculate the correct dosage to be given, if necessary.	☐	☐	______
5. Remove the cap from the container, touching only the outside of the lid.	☐	☐	______
6. Remove the correct dose of medication from the container.	☐	☐	______
7. Greet and identify the patient. Explain the procedure. Ask the patient about medication allergies that might not be noted on the chart.	☐	☐	______
8. Give the medication to the patient.	☐	☐	______
9. Give the patient a glass of water for swallowing the medication unless contraindicated.	☐	☐	______
10. Remain with the patient to be sure that all of the medication is swallowed. Observe any unusual reactions, and report them to the physician. Record any unusual reactions on the patient's chart.	☐	☐	______
11. Wash your hands.	☐	☐	______

☐ **Pass** ☐ **Fail**

Comments

____

____

____

____

Procedure 8-2 Administering Sublingual or Buccal Medications

NAME ______________________ **DATE/TIME** ______________

EVALUATED ______________________ **SCORE** ______________

Goal—To administer a sublingual or buccal medication.

Objectives/Conditions—Upon receiving a physician order to give a sublingual or buccal medication, the student will obtain the appropriate supplies, other items, and the correct medication. The correct medication and dosage will be given either through a sublingual or buccal route.

Outcome—A sublingual or buccal medication is correctly given in accordance with the steps presented in the text.

Equipment and Supplies

Medication
Medication tray
Disposable cup
Physician's instructions

Steps	Y	N	Number of Attempts
1–7. Follow steps 1–7 as described in Procedure 8-1, Administering Oral Medications.	☐	☐	______
8. Administer the medication.	☐	☐	______
9. Remain with the patient to be sure that the medication is *not* swallowed and is allowed to dissolve completely. Do not allow the patient to ingest any food or water until the medication is completely absorbed.	☐	☐	______
10. Observe any unusual reactions, and report them to the physician. Record any unusual reactions on the patient's chart.	☐	☐	______
11. Wash your hands.	☐	☐	______

☐ Pass ☐ Fail

Comments

____

____

____

____

Procedure 8-3 Applying Transdermal Medications

NAME ______________________ **DATE/TIME** ______________

EVALUATED ______________________ **SCORE** ______________

Goal—To apply a transdermal medication.

Objectives/Conditions—Upon receiving a physician order to give a transdermal medication, the student will obtain the appropriate supplies, other items, and the correct medication. The correct medication will be applied transdermally.

Outcome—A transdermal medication is correctly applied in accordance with the steps presented in the text.

Equipment and Supplies

Medication
Medication tray
Physician's order

Steps	Y	N	Number of Attempts
1. Wash your hands.	☐	☐	______
2. Assemble the equipment and supplies.	☐	☐	______
3. Greet and identify the patient. Explain the procedure. Ask the patient about medication allergies that might not be noted on the chart.	☐	☐	______
4. Select the site for administration, and perform any necessary skin preparation. The sites are usually the upper arm, the chest or back surface, or behind the ear; these should be rotated. Ensure that the skin is dry, clean, and free of any irritation. Do not shave areas with excessive hair; trim the hair closely with scissors.	☐	☐	______
5. You may glove at this point. If there is a patch already in place, remove it carefully. If you choose not to glove, do not touch the inside of the patch to avoid absorbing any remaining medication. Discard the used patch in the trash container. Inspect the site for irritation.	☐	☐	______
6. Open the medication package by pulling the two sides apart. Do not touch the area of medication.	☐	☐	______
7. Apply the medicated patch to the patient's skin following the manufacturer's directions. Press the adhesive edges down firmly all around, starting at the center and pressing outward. If the edges do not stick, fasten with paper tape.	☐	☐	______
8. Wash your hands.	☐	☐	______

☐ **Pass** ☐ **Fail**

Comments

____

____

____

____

Procedure 8-4 Applying Topical Medications

NAME ______________________ **DATE/TIME** ______________

EVALUATED ______________________ **SCORE** ______________

Goal—To apply a topical medication.

Objectives/Conditions—Upon receiving a physician order to apply a topical medication, the student will obtain the appropriate supplies, other items, and the correct medication. The correct medication will be applied topically.

Outcome—A topical medication is correctly applied in accordance with the steps presented in the text.

Equipment and Supplies

Medication
Medication tray
Physician's order
Washing solution (optional)
Tongue blade
Large cotton-tipped swab
Gloves
Dressing, bandage, tape (optional)

Steps	Y	N	Number of Attempts
1. Wash your hands.	☐	☐	________
2. Assemble the equipment and supplies. Check the medication label three times.	☐	☐	________
3. Greet and identify the patient. Explain the procedure. Ask the patient about medication allergies that might not be noted on the chart.	☐	☐	________
4. Assess the area to record observations regarding the condition of the skin.	☐	☐	________
5. Put on gloves, in most instances.	☐	☐	________
6. If the area is soiled, clean the skin according to the steps for skin preparation outlined in Procedure 6-4, Performing Skin Preparation and Hair Removal in Chapter 6, Assisting with Minor Office Surgery.	☐	☐	________
7. If old medication remains in the area from a previous treatment, remove it by the same procedure.	☐	☐	________
8. If the lesion requires a dressing and bandage, apply the medication to the dressing using a tongue blade.	☐	☐	________
9. If the medication is to be applied directly to the area, lightly spread it with a tongue blade or a large cotton-tipped swab working from the center of the area outward.	☐	☐	________
10. Use clean technique or medical asepsis if there are no open lesions. Use no touch technique or surgical asepsis if the skin is broken.	☐	☐	________

Steps (Continued)	Y	N	Number of Attempts
11. Bandage if necessary.	☐	☐	______
12. Clean the treatment room, and dispose of equipment and supplies appropriately. Wash your hands.	☐	☐	______

☐ Pass ☐ Fail

Comments

Procedure 8-5 Preparing an Injection

NAME ______________________ **DATE/TIME** ______________

EVALUATED ______________________ **SCORE** ______________

Goal—To prepare an injection.
Objectives/Conditions—When asked to prepare an injection, the student will obtain appropriate equipment, supplies, and the correct medication. An injection is prepared.
Outcome—An injection is correctly prepared in accordance with the steps presented in the text.

Equipment and Supplies

Medication	Appropriate-sized needle and syringe
Medication tray	Physician's instructions
Antiseptic wipes	

Steps	**Y**	**N**	**Number of Attempts**
1. Wash your hands.	☐	☐	______
2. Assemble the equipment and supplies. Be careful to choose the needle and syringe according to the route of administration, type of medication, and patient's size.	☐	☐	______
3. Select the proper medication. Check the expiration date, and check the medication three times: when taking it from the shelf, while drawing it up, and when returning it to the shelf.	☐	☐	______
4. If necessary, calculate the correct dosage to be given.	☐	☐	______
5. Open the sterile syringe/needle package. Assemble if necessary.	☐	☐	______
6. Check to make sure the needle is firmly attached to the syringe by grasping the needle at the hub and turning it clockwise onto the syringe held in the other hand. Remove the needle guard.	☐	☐	______
7. Withdraw the correct amount of medication from the ampule or vial.	☐	☐	______
a. *From an ampule:*			
(1) With the fingertips of one hand, tap the stem of the ampule lightly to remove any medication in or above the arrow neck.	☐	☐	______
(2) Place a piece of gauze around the ampule neck to protect your fingers from broken glass. Grasp the gauze and ampule firmly with the fingers. Snap the stem off the ampule with a quick downward movement of the gauze. Be sure to aim the break away from your face. Set the ampule top aside to discard.	☐	☐	______
(3) Insert the needle lumen below the level of the medication. Withdraw the medication by pulling back on the plunger of the syringe without letting the needle touch the unsterile broken edge of the ampule to avoid contaminating the needle. Withdraw the desired amount of medication; set the ampule aside to dispose of properly.	☐	☐	______

Steps (Continued)	**Y**	**N**	**Number of Attempts**
(4) If there are air bubbles in the syringe, hold it vertically with the needle uppermost, and tap the barrel gently with the fingertips until the air bubbles rise to the top. Draw back on the plunger to admit a small amount of air, then gently push the plunger forward to eject all of the air in the syringe. Do not eject any of the medication if only the required dosage has been drawn up. *Note:* Special needle adapters are available with filters to guard against the possibility of aspirating minute glass particles into the medication to be administered. Discard the adapter needle after drawing up the medication, and attach the appropriate sized needle for the situation to the syringe for the administration of the medication.	☐	☐	______
b. *From a vial:*			
(1) Cleanse the rubber stopper of the vial with the antiseptic wipe to avoid introducing microorganisms into the medication.	☐	☐	______
(2) Pull back on the plunger to aspirate an amount of air equal to the amount of medication to be removed from the vial.	☐	☐	______
(3) Insert the needle through the cleansed center of the stopper and above the level of the medication to prevent foam or bubbles from forming in the medication. Inject the air from the syringe into the vial to avoid forming a vacuum in the vial, which would make withdrawal of the medication difficult.	☐	☐	______
(4) Invert the vial, holding the syringe at eye level. Aspirate the desired amount of medication into the syringe.	☐	☐	______
(5) Remove any air bubbles in the medication within the syringe by gently tapping with the finger tips on the barrel of the syringe held vertically. Remove any air remaining in the syringe by slowly pushing the plunger. Doing this allows the air to flow back into the vial to maintain the equalized pressure.	☐	☐	______
8. Carefully recap the needle.	☐	☐	______
9. Place the syringe with the medication on the medication tray with the physician's instructions. Place an antiseptic wipe on the tray for administering the medication. You are now ready to proceed with administering the specific type of injection ordered by the physician (see Procedures 8-6 to 8-10).	☐	☐	______

☐ **Pass** ☐ **Fail**

Comments

______

______

______

______

Procedure 8-6 Administering an Intradermal Injection

NAME ______________________ DATE/TIME ______________

EVALUATED ______________________ SCORE ______________

Goal—To administer an intradermal injection.

Objectives/Conditions—When asked to administer an intradermal injection, the student will obtain appropriate equipment, supplies, and the correct medication. The student will demonstrate the correct intradermal injection technique.

Outcome—An intradermal injection is administered in accordance with the steps presented in the text.

Equipment and Supplies

Medication
Medication tray
Antiseptic wipe
Appropriate-sized needle and syringe (generally a 1/8-inch 26–28 gauge needle on a tuberculp syringe to administer 0.1–0.2 mL)
Physician's instructions
Gloves

Steps	Y	N	Number of Attempts
1. Prepare the injection according to the steps in Procedure 8-5.	☐	☐	______
2. Greet and identify the patient. Explain the procedure. Ask the patient about medication allergies that might not be noted on the chart.	☐	☐	______
3. Select the appropriate site for the injection. Recommended sites are the anterior forearm and the middle of the back. Make sure the entire site is exposed for safety and accuracy.	☐	☐	______
4. Prepare the site by cleansing with an antiseptic wipe. Use a circular motion starting at the injection site and working outward. Do not touch the site after cleaning. If the site is grossly contaminated, wash it first with soap and water, then clean with an antiseptic wipe.	☐	☐	______
5. Put on gloves.	☐	☐	______
6. Remove the needle guard. Using your nondominant hand, pull the patient's skin taut.	☐	☐	______
7. With the level of the needle facing up, insert the needle at a 10- to 15-degree angle into the upper layer of the skin. When correctly placed for an intradermal injection, the needle will be slightly visible below the surface of the skin. It is not necessary to aspirate when performing an intradermal injection.	☐	☐	______
8. Release the skin held in the nondominant hand and secure the needle hub with the thumb and forefinger. Inject the medication slowly by depressing the plunger. A wheal will form as the medication enters the dermal layer of the skin. Hold the syringe steady for proper administration.	☐	☐	______

Steps (Continued)	Y	N	Number of Attempts
9. Remove the needle from the skin at the same angle at which it was inserted. Gently hold an antiseptic wipe over the site as the needle is withdrawn. Do not press or massage the site.	☐	☐	______
10. Dispose of the syringe and the needle in the approved container. Do not recap the needle. The sharps container should be placed where you have easy access to it after administration of an injection.	☐	☐	______
11. Caution the patient not to massage the site.	☐	☐	______
12. Remove gloves and wash your hands.	☐	☐	______
13. Remain with the patient following the administration of an intradermal injection to observe for any unusual reactions. *Note:* If the patient experiences any unusual reactions, notify the physician immediately.	☐	☐	______
14. Depending on the type of skin test administered, the length of time required for the body tissues to react, and the policies of the medical office, perform one of the following:	☐	☐	______
a. Read the test results. Inspect and palpate the site for the presence and amount of induration.	☐	☐	______
b. Tell the patient when to return (date and time) to the office to have the results read.	☐	☐	______
c. Instruct the patient to read the results at home. Make sure the patient understands the instructions. Have the patient repeat the instructions if necessary.	☐	☐	______

☐ **Pass** ☐ **Fail**

Comments

____

____

____

____

Procedure 8-7 Administering a Tine or Mantoux Test

NAME ______________________ **DATE/TIME** ______________

EVALUATED ______________________ **SCORE** ______________

Goal—To administer a tine or Mantoux test.

Objectives/Conditions—When asked to administer a tine or Mantoux test, the student will obtain appropriate equipment, supplies, and the correct medication. The student will demonstrate the correct techniques for both the tine and the Mantoux test.

Outcome—A tine or Mantoux test is administered in accordance with the steps presented in the text.

Equipment and Supplies

Tine applicator or tuberculin syringe with 1/8–1/2 inch, 26–27 gauge needle with 0.1 mL purified protein derivative
Millimeter ruler
Acetone to wipe or alcohol wipe
Gloves

Steps	Y	N	Number of Attempts
1. Wash your hands.	☐	☐	________
2. For the tine test, obtain the tine applicator. For the Mantoux test, prepare the injection according to the steps in Procedure 8-5.	☐	☐	________
3. Greet and identify the patient. Explain the procedure.	☐	☐	________
4. Assess the area of the forearm about 4 inches below the antecubital area.	☐	☐	________
5. Clean the area with outward, circular strokes with the acetone wipe. Allow to dry.	☐	☐	________
6. Put on gloves.	☐	☐	________
7. Grasp the forearm with the nondominant hand to stretch the skin, secure the site, and make it easier to pierce the skin.	☐	☐	________
a. *For the Mantoux test:* Follow steps 7–9 of Procedure 8-6, Administering an Intradermal Injection.	☐	☐	________
b. *For the tine test:* Uncap the tester and press it into the skin.	☐	☐	________
Hold for 1–2 seconds, release the tension on the skin, and remove the tester.	☐	☐	________
8. Do not massage the site in either method. Cover the site gently and briefly with an alcohol wipe but do not press or wipe.	☐	☐	________
9. Properly care for or dispose of equipment and supplies. Remove gloves and wash your hands.	☐	☐	________

Steps (Continued)	**Y**	**N**	**Number of Attempts**
10. Advise the patient regarding returning for evaluation of the test or give instructions regarding the evaluation card to be completed in 48–72 hours and returned by mail. *Note:* If the patient is to return for evaluation of the test, read the results in a good light with the arm slightly flexed. Palpate from the outside area to the center of induration and measure using a millimeter ruler. Disregard erythema and measure only the area of induration. Record the results.	☐	☐	________

☐ **Pass** ☐ **Fail**

Comments

____

____

____

____

Procedure 8-8 Administering a Subcutaneous Injection

NAME ______________________ **DATE/TIME** ______________

EVALUATED ______________________ **SCORE** ______________

Goal—To administer a subcutaneous injection.

Objectives/Conditions—When asked to administer a subcutaneous injection, the student will obtain appropriate equipment, supplies, and the correct medication. The student will demonstrate the correct subcutaneous injection technique.

Outcome—A subcutaneous injection is administered in accordance with the steps presented in the text.

Equipment and Supplies

Medication
Medication tray
Antiseptic wipe
Appropriate-sized needle and syringe (generally a 1/2–5/8 inch, 24–28 gauge needle on a regular 2–3 mL syringe or tuberculin syringe)
Physician's instructions
Gloves

Steps	Y	N	Number of Attempts
1. Prepare the injection according to the steps in Procedure 8-5.	☐	☐	________
2. Greet and identify the patient. Explain the procedure. Ask the patient about medication allergies that might not be noted on the chart.	☐	☐	________
3. Select the appropriate site for the injection. The upper arm, thigh, back, and abdomen are common sites for subcutaneous injections. Make sure the entire site is exposed for accuracy and safety.	☐	☐	________
4. Put on gloves.	☐	☐	________
5. Prepare the site by cleansing with an antiseptic wipe. Use a circular motion starting at the injection site and working outward. Do not touch the site after cleaning. If the site is grossly contaminated, wash it first with soap and water, then clean with an antiseptic wipe.	☐	☐	________
6. Remove the needle guard. Using the nondominant hand, hold the skin surrounding the injection site in a cushion fashion.	☐	☐	________
7. With a firm motion, insert the needle into the tissue at a 45-degree angle to the skin. Hold the barrel between the thumb and index finger of the dominant hand, and insert the needle up to the hub into the tissue.	☐	☐	________
8. Remove your nondominant hand from the skin.	☐	☐	________
9. With the thumb and forefinger of the nondominant hand on the hub of the needle to hold the syringe steady, pull back on the plunger slightly. If blood appears in the syringe, a vessel has been entered. If this occurs, prepare a new injection and repeat steps 4–9.	☐	☐	________

Steps (Continued)	Y	N	Number of Attempts
10. Inject the medication slowly and steadily by depressing the plunger.	☐	☐	______
11. Place an antiseptic wipe over the injection site, and remove the needle at the same angle at which it was injected.	☐	☐	______
12. Properly dispose of the syringe and needle into an approved sharps container. Do not recap the needle. The sharps container should be placed where you have easy access to it after giving the injection.	☐	☐	______
13. Gently massage the injection site with the antiseptic wipe. Apply pressure to the site and cover with an adhesive bandage if needed. Heparin, sometimes given subcutaneously, is not massaged because it may cause excessive bleeding into the site.	☐	☐	______
14. Remove your gloves and wash your hands.	☐	☐	______
15. Remain with the patient to observe for any unusual reactions. An injection given for allergy desensitization requires that the patient remain in the office for at least 30 minutes to be observed for a reaction. Assist the patient from the examination table if necessary. *Note:* If the patient experiences any unusual reactions, notify the physician immediately.	☐	☐	______

☐ **Pass** ☐ **Fail**

Comments

____

____

____

____

Procedure 8-9 Administering an Intramuscular Injection

NAME ______________________ **DATE/TIME** ______________

EVALUATED ______________________ **SCORE** ______________

Goal—To administer an intramuscular injection.

Objectives/Conditions—When asked to administer an intramuscular injection, the student will obtain appropriate equipment, supplies, and the correct medication. The student will demonstrate the correct intramuscular injection technique.

Outcome—An intramuscular injection is administered in accordance with the steps presented in the text.

Equipment and Supplies

Medication
Medication tray
Antiseptic wipe
Appropriate-sized needle and syringe (generally 1/2 inch, 20–23 gauge regular 2–5 mL syringe for the injection of up to 3 mL per site)
Physician's instructions
Gloves

Steps	Y	N	Number of Attempts
1. Prepare the injection according to the steps in Procedure 8-5.	☐	☐	________
2. Greet and identify the patient. Explain the procedure. Ask the patient about medication allergies that might not be noted on the chart.	☐	☐	________
3. Select the appropriate site for the injection (see Figs. 8-14 through 8-18) and the appropriate syringe.	☐	☐	________
4. Prepare the site by cleansing with an antiseptic wipe. Use a circular motion starting at the injection site and working outward. Do not touch the site after cleaning. If the site is grossly contaminated, wash it first with soap and water, then clean with an antiseptic wipe.	☐	☐	________
5. Put on gloves.	☐	☐	________
6. Remove the needle guard. Pull the skin taut over the injection site using the thumb and index fingers of the nondominant hand. *Note:* Patients with meager muscle mass may require that you grasp the muscle and "bunch" it to ensure that the medication is inserted as deeply into the area as possible.	☐	☐	________
7. Hold the syringe like a dart. Using a quick, firm motion, insert the needle at a 90-degree angle to the skin.	☐	☐	________
8. With the thumb and forefinger of the nondominant hand, hold the syringe steady, pull back slightly on the plunger with the dominant hand. If blood appears in the syringe, you must prepare a new injection and repeat steps 4–8.	☐	☐	________
9. Slowly inject the medication by steadily depressing the plunger of the syringe.	☐	☐	________

Steps (Continued)	**Y**	**N**	**Number of Attempts**
10. Place an antiseptic wipe over the injection site. Remove the needle quickly and at the same angle at which it was inserted.	☐	☐	________
11. Properly dispose of the needle and syringe in an approved sharps container. Do not recap the needle. The sharps container should be placed where you have easy access to it after the injection has been administered.	☐	☐	________
12. Gently massage the injection site with an antiseptic wipe. Apply pressure to the site and cover with an adhesive bandage if needed.	☐	☐	________
13. Remove gloves and wash your hands.	☐	☐	________
14. Remain with the patient to observe for any unusual reactions. Assist the patient off the examination table if necessary. *Note:* If the patient experiences any unusual reaction, notify the physician immediately.	☐	☐	________

☐ **Pass** ☐ **Fail**

Comments

____

____

____

____

Procedure 8-10 Administering an Intramuscular Injection Using the Z-Track Method

NAME ______________________ **DATE/TIME** ______________

EVALUATED ______________________ **SCORE** ______________

Goal—To administer an intramuscular injection using the Z-track method.

Objectives/Conditions—When asked to administer an intramuscular injection using the Z-track method, the student will obtain appropriate equipment, supplies, and the correct medication. The student will demonstrate the correct intramuscular Z-track technique.

Outcome—An intramuscular injection using the Z-track method is administered in accordance with the steps presented in the text.

Equipment and Supplies

Medication
Medication tray
Antiseptic wipe
Appropriate-sized needle and syringe
Physician's instructions
Gloves

Steps	Y	N	Number of Attempts
1–5. Follow steps 1–5 as described in Procedure 8-9, Administering an Intramuscular Injection. *Note:* The ventrogluteal, vastus lateralis, and dorsogluteal sites work well for the Z-track method; the deltoid does not.	☐	☐	______
6. Remove the needle guard. Rather than pulling the skin taut or grasping the tissue as you would for an intramuscular injection, pull the top layer of skin to the side and hold it with the nondominant hand.	☐	☐	______
7. Insert the needle to the hub at a 90-degree angle in a quick, dartlike motion.	☐	☐	______
8. With the side of the nondominant hand holding the displaced skin, grasp the hub of the needle with the thumb and forefinger and aspirate by withdrawing the plunger slightly with the dominant hand. If no blood appears, push the plunger in slowly and steadily. Count to 10 before withdrawing the needle.	☐	☐	______
9. Cover the area with an antiseptic wipe. Withdraw the needle and release the skin. Most Z-track medications must not be massaged to avoid forcing the medication into upper tissues. Check the manufacturer's guidelines.	☐	☐	______
10. Properly dispose of the needle and syringe in an approved sharps container. Do not recap the needle. The sharps container should be placed where you have easy access to it after the injection has been administered.	☐	☐	______

Steps (Continued)	Y	N	Number of Attempts
11. Remove gloves and wash your hands.	☐	☐	______
12. Remain with the patient to observe for any unusual reactions. Assist the patient off of the examination table if necessary. *Note:* If the patient experiences any unusual reaction, notify the physician immediately.	☐	☐	______

☐ Pass ☐ Fail

Comments

____

____

____

____

9

Introduction to Anatomy and Physiology

COMPETENCY PRACTICE

Vocabulary Assessment

Matching

Match the term in Part 1 with correct definition in Part 2.

PART 1

1. medial
2. proximal
3. deep
4. superficial
5. distal
6. sagittal
7. frontal

PART 2

a. _____ plane divides body into left and right
b. _____ further from the point of origin
c. _____ far from the surface
d. _____ away from the midline, to the side
e. _____ close to the midline of the body
f. _____ plane dividing body into front and back
g. _____ close to the point of origin

Definitions

Define the following key terms.

1. anatomical position

____

____

____

2. anatomy

____

____

____

3. element

____

____

____

4. physiology

5. planes

6. quadrants

7. systems

Critical Thinking

1. Explain positive and negative feedback. Give an example of each.

2. Identify and describe the levels of organization of the body in ascending order.

Case Studies

1. Jack Lee, aged 12, is being seen for a laceration on his left forearm. He hears you ask another medical assistant to set up a minor surgical tray for a 2-cm long, deep laceration, located proximal to the elbow and the medial aspect of the posterior left forearm. He asks you what those terms mean. What will you tell the patient?

2. Mrs. Smith, aged 45, calls the office and requests an appointment because of a complaint of pain. As you take a history, Mrs. Smith points to the area of discomfort, under her right rib area. She states that she has been in pain for about a week, especially after meals. She has experienced nausea but no diarrhea. What is the medical term for the area where her pain is? Why does this area have a specific name?

CHARTING EXERCISE

Using Case Study #2, write a chart note documenting the reason for the patient's visit to the physician.

Document on the Patient's Chart:

- Date and time
- Notification of physician
- Patient complaints/concerns
- Patient education
- Your signature

Date/Time	Conditions/Lab Results Patient Communication

Basic Writing Activities

Skill Drills

1. List five cavities of the body.

____

____

____

2. List the organs contained in the thoracic cavity.

____

____

____

3. Describe the body when it is in an anatomical position.

____

____

____

4. List the abdominal regions.

____

____

____

Fill-in-the-Blanks

1. The fundamental unit of all living tissue is the ______________.

2. ______________ are made up of a collection of similar cells and their supporting structures acting together to perform a particular function.

3. The abdominal cavity is made up of ______________ abdominal regions.

4. ______________ is an increase in a body function in response to a stimulus.

5. All cells, no matter the shape, size, or function, have three main parts: the ______________, ______________, and ______________.

6. The ______________ is the smallest component of an ______________ that contains the physical properties of that element.

Innovative Activities

Labeling

Identify the seven cavities of the body.

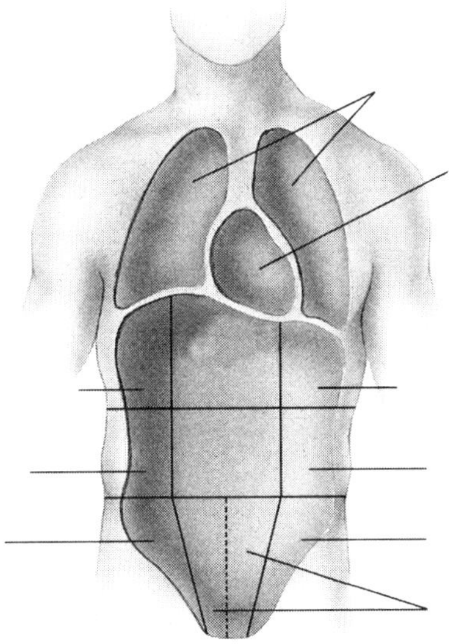

10

Assisting With Diagnostic and Therapeutic Procedures Associated With the Integumentary System

COMPETENCY PRACTICE

Vocabulary Assessment

Matching

Match the definition in Part 1 with the correct term in Part 2.

PART 1

1. small, flat skin discoloration
2. small fluid-filled sac
3. large fluid-filled sac
4. pus-filled sac
5. deep infection of a hair follicle

PART 2

a. _____ furuncle

b. _____ bullae

c. _____ pustule

d. _____ vesicles

d. _____ macule

Definitions

Define each of the following terms.

1. abscess

____

____

2. comedo

____

____

3. fissure

____

____

4. nodule

____

____

5. urticaria

____

____

6. dermatophytosis

____

____

Critical Thinking

1. Keloids, an overproduction of scar tissue, occur as a complication of wound healing. What segment of the population is most frequently affected and where are the common sites on the body?

2. Bedridden patients are at risk for developing decubiti. How do decubitus ulcers form, and what parts of the bedridden body are most at risk? What actions can be taken to reduce the risk of decubiti developing?

Case Studies

1. Miss Smith is a 23-year-old female who is concerned about the appearance of a draining wound on her left anterior thigh. Dr. White will be examining Miss Smith and will probably order a wound culture. How will you prepare Miss Smith for the examination?

2. Mr. Connors is a 70-year-old man with a lesion on his left leg. Dr. Greene has prescribed warm compresses three times a day. Mrs. Connors will be applying the compresses and is anxious to do everything correctly. How would you educate Mr. and Mrs. Connors about such issues as purpose, performance, and expected outcomes of the compresses? What precautions or danger signs would you explain to Mr. and Mrs. Connors?

CHARTING EXERCISE

Using the situation described in Case Study #1, write a narrative chart note describing your interaction with patient, including the collection of the wound culture.

Document on the Patient's Chart:

- Date and time
- Notification of physician
- Patient complaints/concerns
- Patient education
- Your signature

Date/Time	Conditions/Lab Results Patient Communication

Basic Writing Activities

Skill Drills

1. List the three basic layers of the skin.

2. Identify and explain three functions of the integumentary system.

____

____

____

3. What are the four most common causes of urticaria (hives)?

____

____

____

4. List four items that should be included in an emergency cart or tray when a patient is receiving allergy testing.

____

____

____

Fill-in-the-Blanks

1. The most common malignant tumor of the skin of whites is ______________________.
2. A sunscreen with at least a ______________________ SPF (sun protective factor) is considered good protection in blocking ultraviolet rays.
3. Sudoriferous glands are also known as ______________________ glands.
4. Vitamin ______________________ is necessary for the absorption of calcium and phosphorus from the small intestine.
5. Impetigo may by caused by ______________________ or ______________________ organisms, types of bacteria commonly implicated in skin disease.

Innovative Activities

Create an educational brochure, appropriate for a medical office, on pediculosis capitis.

COMPETENCY EVALUATION CHECKLIST

Procedure 10-1 Applying Cold

NAME ______________________ **DATE/TIME** ______________

EVALUATED ______________________ **SCORE** ______________

Goal—To apply cold.
Objectives/Conditions—When asked to demonstrate the correct method of applying cold, the student will obtain appropriate equipment and supplies and correctly apply cold.
Outcome—A cold application is demonstrated, using correct techniques and in accordance with the steps presented in the text.

Equipment and Supplies

Ice bag or ice collar or disposable cold pack
Cover
Ice chips or small cubes
Gauze or tape

Steps	Y	N	Number of Attempts
1. Wash your hands.	☐	☐	______
2. Assemble the equipment and supplies, checking the bag or collar for leaks. If using a commercial cold pack, read the manufacturer's directions.	☐	☐	______
3. Fill the container about two-thirds full. Press it flat on a surface to expell excess air from within. Seal the container.	☐	☐	______
4. Cover the bag.	☐	☐	______
5. Greet and identify the patient. Explain the procedure.	☐	☐	______
6. If using a commercial pack, activate it now.	☐	☐	______
7. Assess the area.	☐	☐	______
8. Ensure the patient's comfort.	☐	☐	______
9. Secure the appliance with gauze or tape.	☐	☐	______
10. Apply no longer than 30 minutes.	☐	☐	______
11. Assess the area for mottling, pallor, redness, or pain.	☐	☐	______
12. If the treatment is to be reapplied, wait 1 hour.	☐	☐	______
13. Properly care for or dispose of equipment and supplies. Wash your hands.	☐	☐	______

☐ Pass ☐ Fail

Comments

____

____

____

____

Procedure 10-2 Applying a Warm or Cold Compress

NAME ______________________ **DATE/TIME** ______________

EVALUATED ______________________ **SCORE** ______________

Goal—To apply a warm or cold compress.

Objectives/Conditions—When asked to demonstrate the correct methods of applying a warm or cold compress, the student will obtain appropriate equipment and supplies and correctly apply a warm or cold compress.

Outcome—A warm or cold compress is demonstrated, using correct techniques and in accordance with the steps presented in the text.

Equipment and Supplies

Appropriate solution, warmed or cooled to recommended temperature
Absorbent material of the physician's choice
Waterproof barriers and insulators
Thermometer
Hot water bottle or cold pack
Clean or sterile basin
Sterile gloves or sterile transfer forceps, if appropriate

Steps	Y	N	Number of Attempts
1. Wash your hands. *Note:* If an open wound is present, observe surgical asepsis as outlined in Chap. 6, Assisting With Minor Office Surgery.	☐	☐	______
2. Assemble the equipment and supplies. Pour the solution into the basin. Check the temperature of the solution.	☐	☐	______
3. Greet and identify the patient. Explain the procedure.	☐	☐	______
4. Ensure patient comfort and privacy.	☐	☐	______
5. Protect the undersurface and clothing with waterproof barriers.	☐	☐	______
6. Put on gloves. Press or wring out excess mositure from the absorbent material. If using sterile procedure, this may be done with sterile gloves or with two sterile transfer forceps.	☐	☐	______
7. Touch the compress to the area lightly, and observe the patient's reaction or ask for a response.	☐	☐	______
8. Check the surface of the skin.	☐	☐	______
9. Gently arrange the compress over the area and conform the material to the patient's contours. Insulate the compress with waterproof barriers.	☐	☐	______
10. Check frequently for moisture and temperature. Hot water bottles or ice packs may be used to maintain the temperature.	☐	☐	______

Steps (Continued)	Y	N	Number of Attempts
11. Discontinue after 30 minutes. Wait 1 hour before reapplying.	☐	☐	______
12. Discard disposable materials, and appropriately disinfect reusable equipment. Wash your hands.	☐	☐	______

☐ **Pass** ☐ **Fail**

Comments

______

______

______

______

Procedure 10-3 Using a Hot Water Bottle or Commercial Hot Pack

NAME ______________________ **DATE/TIME** ______________

EVALUATED ______________________ **SCORE** ______________

Goal—To use a hot water bottle or commercial hot pack.

Objectives/Conditions—When asked to demonstrate the correct methods of using a hot water bottle or a commercial hot pack, the student will obtain appropriate equipment and supplies and correctly use a hot water bottle or commercial hot pack.

Outcomes—A hot water bottle or commercial hot pack is used correctly and in accordance with the steps presented in the text.

Equipment and Supplies

Hot water bottle or commercial hot pack
Cover
Thermometer

Steps	Y	N	Number of Attempts
1. Wash your hands.	☐	☐	________
2. Assemble equipment, being sure to check the hot water bottle for leaks.	☐	☐	________
3. Fill bottle about two-thirds full with water at appropriate temperature. Check temperature with thermometer.	☐	☐	________
4. Place the bottle on a flat surface with the opening up and "burp" it by pressing out the excess air.	☐	☐	________
5. If using a commercial hot pack, follow the manufacturer's directions for activating it.	☐	☐	________
6. Wrap and secure the pack or bottle before placing on the patient's skin.	☐	☐	________
7. Greet and identify the patient. Explain the procedure.	☐	☐	________
8. If continuous heat has been ordered, follow the physician's instructions; otherwise, remove after 30 minutes. Assess the area every 10 minutes.	☐	☐	________
9. Report pallor (an indication of rebound), excessive redness (indicates temperature may be too high for this lesion), swelling (indicates that capillary permeability may contribute to tissue damage).	☐	☐	________
10. Caution the patient that the body will adapt to the temperature and that it is not necessary to increase continually the temperature to achieve maximum benefits.	☐	☐	________

☐ Pass ☐ Fail

Comments

____

____

____

____

Procedure 10-4 Assisting With Therapeutic Soaks

NAME ______________________ **DATE/TIME** ______________

EVALUATED ______________________ **SCORE** ______________

Goal—To assist with a therapeutic soak.

Objectives/Conditions—When asked to assist with a therapeutic soak, the student will obtain appropriate equipment and supplies and correctly demonstrate how to assist with this procedure.

Outcomes—Assisting with therapeutic soaks is performed in accordance with the steps presented in the text.

Equipment and Supplies

Container large enough to contain the part to be soaked comfortably
Towels (for padding surfaces and drying the part)
Solution
Thermometer

Steps	Y	N	Number of Attempts
1. Wash your hands.	☐	☐	______
2. Assemble the equipment and supplies.	☐	☐	______
3. Fill the container with the solution, and check the temperature with the thermometer. (The proper temperature is usually at no more than 110°F [about 45°C] because of the large surface involved and the possibility of blood pressure changes with vasodilation or vasoconstriction.)	☐	☐	______
4. Greet and identify the patient. Explain the procedure.	☐	☐	______
5. Slowly lower the part into the container and check for the patient's reaction. Arrange the part comfortably and in easy alignment. (The basin should be large enough to immerse the entire limb.) Check for pressure areas and pad the edges. The bottom may also be padded for comfort.	☐	☐	______
6. Soak for the prescribed period of time.	☐	☐	______
7. Check every 5–10 minutes for the proper temperature. If additional water or solution must be added to maintain the temperature, remove a quantity of the solution. With your hand acting as a shield between the patient and the stream of solution, add the required amount and swirl it quickly through the container.	☐	☐	______
8. Soak for the prescribed time, usually 15–20 minutes.	☐	☐	______
9. Carefully dry the part.	☐	☐	______
10. Assess the area.	☐	☐	______
11. Properly care for or dispose of equipment and supplies. Wash your hands.	☐	☐	______

☐ Pass ☐ Fail

Comments

____

____

____

____

11

Assisting With Diagnostic and Therapeutic Procedures Associated With the Musculoskeletal System

COMPETENCY PRACTICE

Vocabulary Assessment

Matching

Match the definition in Part 1 with the correct term in Part 2.

PART 1

1. longest, strongest, and heaviest bone in the body
2. shoulder blade
3. knee cap
4. bones of the fingers
5. bones of the hand
6. cheekbones
7. bone cells

PART 2

a. phalanges
b. zygomatic bones
c. metacarpals
d. femur
e. osteocytes
f. patella
g. scapula

Definitions

Write a term for each of the following definitions.

1. slightly moveable joints

____

2. any muscle that opposes the action of the prime mover to balance movement

____

3. repair a joint

____

4. abnormal shortening of muscles around a joint caused by atrophy of the muscles and resulting in flexion and fixation

____

5. muscles that work together for more efficient movement

____

6. instrument used to measure the angle of joints for range of motion

___

7. the process of recording electrical nerve transmission in skeletal muscles

___

Critical Thinking

1. Describe two different kinds of crutches and why one may be favored over the other.

___
___
___

2. What can cause a herniated disk? What are the symptoms?

___
___
___

Case Studies

1. On 10/28/99, Scotty Wright, aged 9, fell off a slide and broke his left arm. The fracture was reduced and a long arm cast applied. At 10:20 a.m. you note that the fingers on Scotty's left hand are warm to touch and pink in color. You fit Scotty with a triangle sling. While waiting to talk to the physician, Scotty's mother asks you how bones heal and why it is important that Scotty wear a sling. What can you tell this patient's mother regarding healing fractures and the need to wear a sling?

___
___
___

2. Mr. Jones has tendonitis of the right arm. After his examination, Dr. Marks asks you to schedule a return appointment in 6 weeks and also give Mr. Jones a patient education brochure on tendonitis. What information will be contained in this brochure?

___
___
___

CHARTING EXERCISE

With regard to Case Study #1, write a narrative chart note describing your interaction with Scotty and his mother.

Document on the Patient's Chart:

- Date and time
- Notification of physician
- Patient complaints/concerns
- Patient education
- Your signature

Date/Time	Conditions/Lab Results Patient Communication

Basic Writing Activities

Skill Drills

1. List and describe the five types of bones.

___
___
___

2. List and describe three abnormal curvatures of the spine.

___
___
___

3. Name and describe four different types of fractures.

___
___
___

Short Answer Questions

1. ______________________ is a degenerative disorder affecting the cartilage underlying the kneecaps.
2. Poorly fitting shoes may cause the following foot deformities:

   ____

   ____

   ____

3. Differentiate between osteoarthritis and rheumatoid arthritis.

   ____

   ____

   ____

4. Identify the part of the body affected by each of the following conditions:
   a. plantar fascitis

   ____

   b. carpal tunnel syndrome

   ____

   c. Dupuytren's contracture

   ____

Innovative Activities

Labeling

Identify the various joint motions.

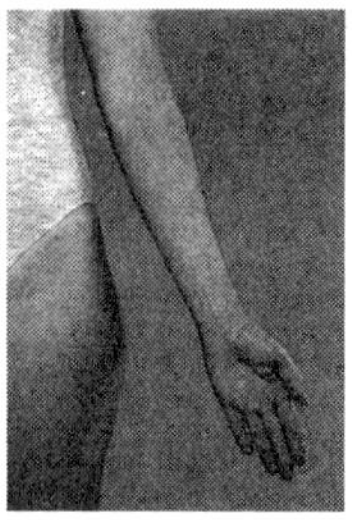
A

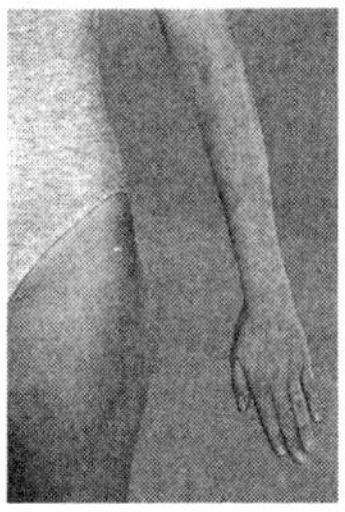
B

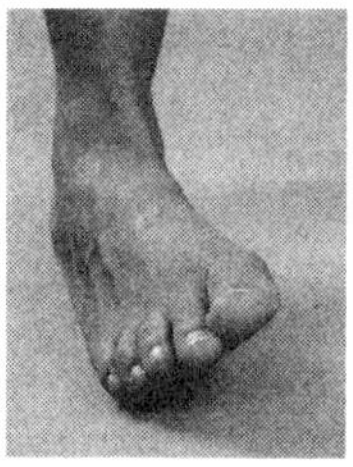
C

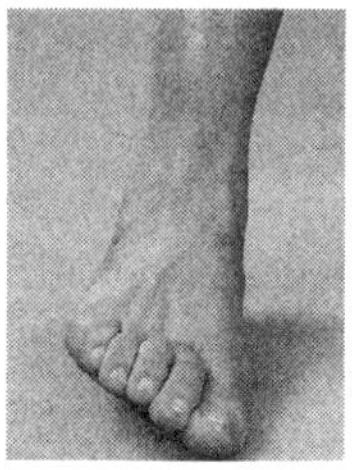
D

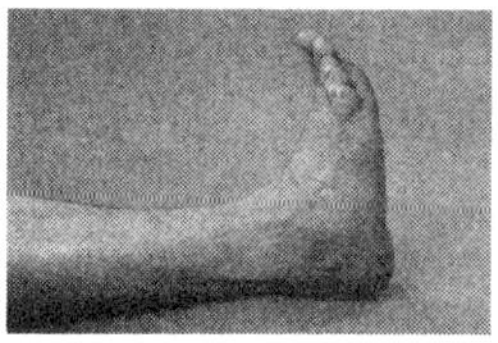
E

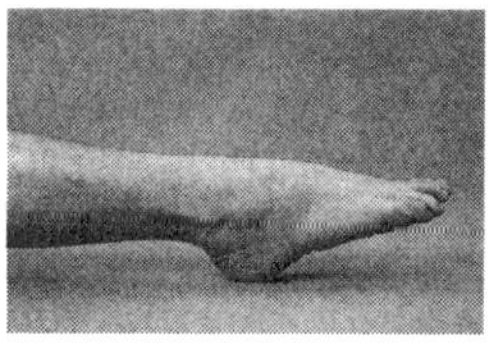
F

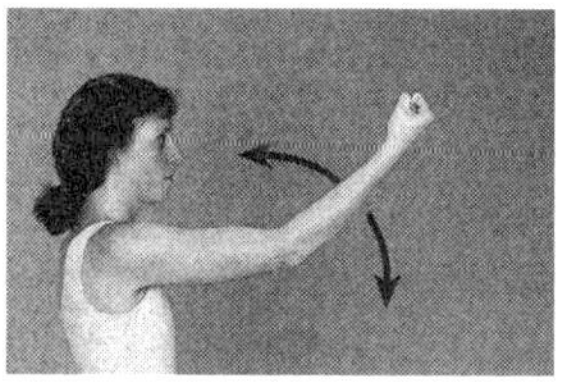
G

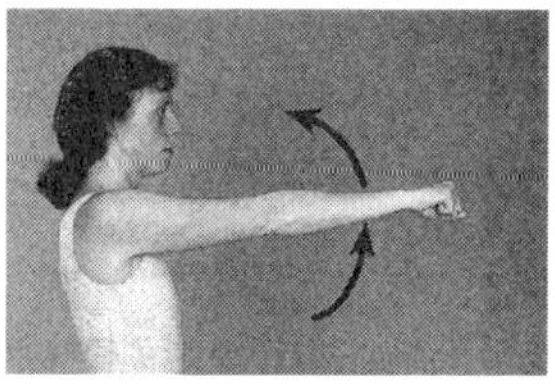
H

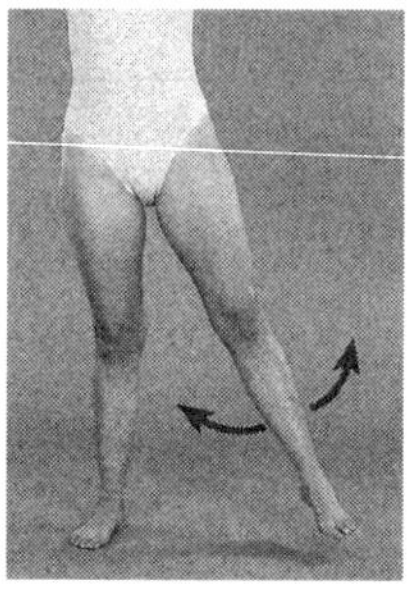
I

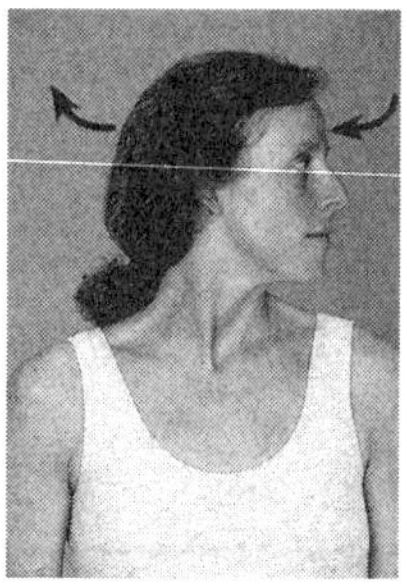
J

A. ______________________

B. ______________________

C. ______________________

D. ______________________

E. ______________________

F. ______________________

G. ______________________

H. ______________________

I. ______________________

J. ______________________

COMPETENCY EVALUATION CHECKLIST

Procedure 11-1 Assisting With Cast Application

NAME ______________________ **DATE/TIME** ______________

EVALUATED ______________________ **SCORE** ______________

Goal—To assist with cast application.
Objectives/Conditions—When given the equipment and supplies listed in the text, the student will assist with cast application.
Outcome—The student will assist with cast application in accordance with steps in the text.

Equipment and Supplies

Tubular soft stockinette fabric, sized to fit the limb
Roller padding/sheet wadding
Casting material, sized to fit the limb
Bucket of cold or tepid water
Plaster cast knife
Utility gloves for physician and assistant

Steps	**Y**	**N**	**Number of Attempts**
1. Wash your hands.	☐	☐	______
2. Assemble the equipment.	☐	☐	______
3. Greet and identify the patient. Explain the procedure and answer any questions.	☐	☐	______
4. Assess the need for size and lengths of fabric stocking, cotton padding, and casting material.	☐	☐	______
5. At the physician's instructions, glove with the heavy utility gloves and begin to soak the casting material in the water. Remove the material when no more bubbles rise from the roll. Do not wring the roll; press the excess water from the roll, and pull free one corner of the first layer of the roll.	☐	☐	______
6. Pass the cast knife to the physician at the completion of the procedure to trim away rough edges of the material.	☐	☐	______
7. Educate the patient regarding cast care for the type of cast applied. Ask for and answer any questions.	☐	☐	______
8. Help the patient reclothe if clothing has been removed for the procedure.	☐	☐	______
9. Care for and properly dispose of equipment and supplies. Wash your hands.	☐	☐	______

☐ **Pass** ☐ **Fail**

Comments

____

____

____

____

Procedure 11-2 Applying a Triangular Arm Sling

NAME ______________________ **DATE/TIME** ______________

EVALUATED ______________________ **SCORE** ______________

Goal—To apply a triangular arm sling.

Objectives/Conditions—When given the equipment and supplies listed in the text, the student will apply a triangular arm sling.

Outcome—The student will apply a triangular arm sling in accordance with steps in the text.

Equipment and Supplies

Sling as ordered by the physician
Pins

Steps	**Y**	**N**	**Number of Attempts**
1. Wash your hands.	☐	☐	______
2. Assemble the equipment.	☐	☐	______
3. Greet and identify the patient. Explain the procedure and ask for questions.	☐	☐	______
4. Position the affected limb with the hand at slightly less than a 90-degree angle so that the fingers are higher than the elbow.	☐	☐	______
5. Place the triangle with the uppermost corner at the shoulder on the unaffected side (extend the corner across the nape), the middle angle at the elbow of the affected side, and the final lowermost corner pointing toward the foot on the unaffected side.	☐	☐	______
6. Bring the lowermost corner up to meet the upper corner at the side of the neck, never at the back of the neck.	☐	☐	______
7. Tie or pin the sling. Secure the elbow by fitting any extra fabric neatly around the limb and pinning it.	☐	☐	______
8. Check the patient's comfort level and distal extremity circulation.	☐	☐	______
9. Wash your hands.	☐	☐	______

☐ **Pass** ☐ **Fail**

Comments

____

____

____

____

Procedure 11-3 Measure a Patient for Axillary Crutches

NAME ______________________ **DATE/TIME** ______________

EVALUATED ______________________ **SCORE** ______________

Goal—To measure a patient for axillary crutches.

Objectives/Conditions—When given the equipment and supplies listed in the text, the student will measure a patient for axillary crutches.

Outcome—The student will measure a patient for axillary crutches in accordance with steps in the text.

Equipment and Supplies

Crutches with safety tips
Pad for the axillae and hand rests, as needed
Tools to tighten bolts

Steps	Y	N	Number of Attempts
1. Wash your hands.	☐	☐	______
2. Assemble the equipment.	☐	☐	______
3. Greet and identify the patient. Explain the procedure.	☐	☐	______
4. Ensure that the patient is wearing low-heeled shoes with safety soles.	☐	☐	______
5. Have the patient stand erect. Support the patient as needed.	☐	☐	______
6. Have the patient hold the crutches naturally with the tips about 2 inches in front of and 4–6 inches to the side of the feet. This is called the tripod position, and all crutch gaits start from this position (see Procedure 11-4: Teaching a Patient Crutch Gaits).	☐	☐	______
7. Using the tools as needed, adjust the crutches to the patient's height:	☐	☐	______
a. Remove the wing nut and bolt, and move the extensions.	☐	☐	______
b. Ensure that the axillary bar is about 2 fingerbreadths below the patient's axilla.	☐	☐	______
c. Tighten the bolts for safety when the proper height is reached.	☐	☐	______
8. Adjust the handgrips.	☐	☐	______
a. Raise or lower the bar along the shaft of the crutch.	☐	☐	______
b. Check the adjustment. Crutches are properly adjusted when the patient's elbow is at a 30-degree angle when the bar is gripped and two fingers can be inserted at the axilla.	☐	☐	______
c. Tighten the bolts for safety.	☐	☐	______

Steps (Continued)	Y	N	Number of Attempts
9. If needed, pad axillary bars and handgrips with soft material to prevent friction.	☐	☐	________
10. Properly care for or dispose of equipment and supplies. Wash your hands.	☐	☐	________

☐ **Pass** ☐ **Fail**

Comments

____

____

____

____

Procedure 11-4 Instruct a Patient in the Use of Various Crutch Gaits

NAME ______________________ **DATE/TIME** ______________

EVALUATED ______________________ **SCORE** ______________

Goal—To instruct a patient in the use of various crutch gaits.

Objectives/Conditions—When given the equipment and supplies listed in the text, the student will instruct a patient in the use of various crutch gaits.

Outcome—The student will instruct a patient in the use of various crutch gaits in accordance with the steps in the text.

Steps	Y	N	Number of Attempts
1. Wash your hands.	☐	☐	______
2. Have the patient stand up from a chair. To do this, the patient holds both crutches on the affected side, then slides to the edge of the chair. The patient pushes down on the chair arm on the unaffected side, then pushes to stand. Weight should be rested on the crutches until balance is restored.	☐	☐	______
3. Ensure that the crutches are in the tripod position.	☐	☐	______
4. Have the patient begin the appropriate gait.	☐	☐	______
a. *Three-point gait*	☐	☐	______
b. *Two-point gait*	☐	☐	______
c. *Four-point gait*	☐	☐	______
d. *Swing-through gait*	☐	☐	______
e. *Swing-to gait*	☐	☐	______
5. Wash your hands.	☐	☐	______

☐ Pass ☐ Fail

Comments

____

____

____

____

Procedure 11-5 Transfer a Patient To and From a Wheelchair

NAME ______________________ **DATE/TIME** ______________

EVALUATED ______________________ **SCORE** ______________

Goal—To transfer a patient to and from a wheelchair.

Objectives/Conditions—When given the equipment and supplies listed in the text, the student will transfer a patient to and from a wheelchair.

Outcome—The student will transfer a patient to and from a wheelchair in accordance with the steps in the text.

Equipment and Supplies

Wheelchair
Transfer belt (optional, but preferred)
Sliding board (optional)

Steps	Y	N	Number of Attempts
1. Wash your hands.	☐	☐	______
2. Explain to both the patient and caregiver how you will facilitate the transfer and how they both may help.	☐	☐	______
3. Organize the setting to ensure the shortest transfer distance possible and ease of maneuvering. If the wheelchair is placed facing the direction the patient either is facing or will need to face, there will be no need to turn the patient.	☐	☐	______
4. Align the wheelchair as close as possible to the point of transfer at either a 45-degree angle or parallel to the patient, preferably on the patient's strongest side. Lock the wheels, and raise the foot rests.	☐	☐	______
5. Assist the patient into position as needed.	☐	☐	______
a. From a vehicle: Standing at the patient's side, slide one arm under his or her thighs, and brace the patient's shoulders with your other arm. In one smooth movement, turn the patient in the seat until his or her feet are toward the ground.	☐	☐	______
b. From the table: With one arm under the patient's shoulders, assist him or her to sit. Help the patient to slide to the end of the table until his or her feet are on the table step. You may require assistance if the patient cannot step down.	☐	☐	______
Note: To assist the patient into the vehicle or onto the table, reverse the procedure.	☐	☐	______
6. Help the patient put on a transfer belt. Secure it snugly.	☐	☐	______
7. Grasp the transfer belt at the back by reaching around the patient's body, or reach under the patient's arms and place your hands on his or her chest wall, not his axilla.	☐	☐	______

Steps (Continued)	Y	N	Number of Attempts
8. Have the patient grasp your shoulders, or have him reach with one hand for the far chair arm for partial support while grasping your shoulder with the other.	☐	☐	______
9. Brace your feet apart with your right foot slightly forward. The patient's foot placement should mirror yours.	☐	☐	______
10. Keep your spine straight. Flex your knees and hips, and brace your knees against the patient's knees. Grasp the transfer belt or tighten your grip on the patient.	☐	☐	______
11. Rock the patient back and forth to an agreed upon count of three. At the signal, encourage the patient to straighten his or her knees and hips. If possible, have the patient push off with the back foot.	☐	☐	______
12. As you straighten, rock your weight onto your back foot, and pivot the patient with his or her back to the destination. Keep your knees against the patient's knees. Support the patient in this position for a moment until balance is restored.	☐	☐	______
13. Have the patient step back to the chair (table or other seat), and grasp the arms of the chair or other surface while you continue to provide stability with your knees against the patient's.	☐	☐	______
14. Shift your weight to your forward foot as the patient lowers to the sitting position.	☐	☐	______
15. Have the patient sit well back into the seat. If in the wheelchair, lower the foot rests and help the patient position his or her feet. If you are to push the patient, make sure the patient's hands are in his or her lap.	☐	☐	______

☐ **Pass** ☐ **Fail**

Comments

____

____

____

____

12

Assisting With Diagnostic and Therapeutic Procedures Associated With the Neurologic System

COMPETENCY PRACTICE

Vocabulary Assessment

Matching

Match the definitions in Part 1 with the correct term in Part 2.

PART 1

1. fundamental functioning units of the nervous system
2. conducts impulses toward the cell body
3. contains the nucleus
4. contains the organelles of the cell
5. transmits impulses away from the cell body
6. fatty insulation formed by Schwann cells
7. junction of two neurons

PART 2

a. _____ cytoplasm

b. _____ neuron

c. _____ axon

d. _____ dendrite

e. _____ cell body

f. _____ synapse

g. _____ myelin sheath

Word Scramble

Unscramble the following medical terms.

1. nops

____

2. lucis

____

3. ruincam

____

4. maticuono

____

5. drachonia

____

Critical Thinking

1. What is the goal of long-term care for patients with spinal cord injuries? List several possible complications.

____

____

____

2. Explain the reflex arc and how it is tested during routine office examinations.

____

____

____

Case Studies

1. George Mendoza, aged 50, is the CEO of a large company. He ingests large amounts coffee and smokes at least one pack of cigarettes per day. He is seeing Dr. Montgomery today at 3:30 p.m. for a complaint of a sudden onset of a "terrible headache on the left side of his head," and "nausea." During the initial history, he complains that the bright lights in the examination room hurt his eyes. You take the patient's vital signs and find that the temperature is 99° F, pulse is 88, respirations are 24, and blood pressure is 138/86. Dr. Montgomery diagnoses the condition as a migraine headache. You medicate the patient, according to the physician's order, and instruct him to rest in the darkened, quiet examination room for a half hour. At 4:40 p.m., the patient's wife arrives to pick him up. On the way out, Mr. Mendoza asks you, "what causes a migraine, anyway?" and "what other symptoms are possible?" How will you educate this patient to the possible causes and symptoms related to migraine headaches?

____

____

____

____

2. Georgia Winters is going through diagnostic testing to determine whether or not she has epilepsy. She has an appointment in your office this afternoon for some blood tests. When she arrives you show her to a room, and while you prepare to draw her blood she asks you about medications for epilepsy and whether, if it turns out that she does have epilepsy, she will ever be able to drive again. How will you respond to this patient?

____

____

____

____

CHARTING EXERCISE

With regard to Case Study #1, write a chart note detailing your interaction with the patient, including medication administration and patient teaching.

Document on the Patient's Chart:

- Date and time
- Notification of physician
- Patient complaints/concerns
- Patient education
- Your signature

Date/Time	Conditions/Lab Results Patient Communication

Basic Writing Activities

Skill Drills

1. Identify the three main components of the brain and list their individual functions.

____

____

____

2. List and explain three types of paralysis.

____

____

____

3. Identify six infectious diseases that involve the nervous system.

____

____

____

4. Explain the physical and emotional effects of two degenerative nervous system disorders.

____

____

____

Fill-in-the-Blanks

1. ________________________ nerves conduct impulses away from the brain.
2. ________________________ nerves conduct impulses to the brain.
3. Dopamine is a ________________________ and is essential for controlling body movement and facial expressions.
4. The ________________________ nervous system is involved with nonemergency functions.
5. Tetanus is commonly called ____________________.

Innovative Activities

Labeling

Identify each neuron part.

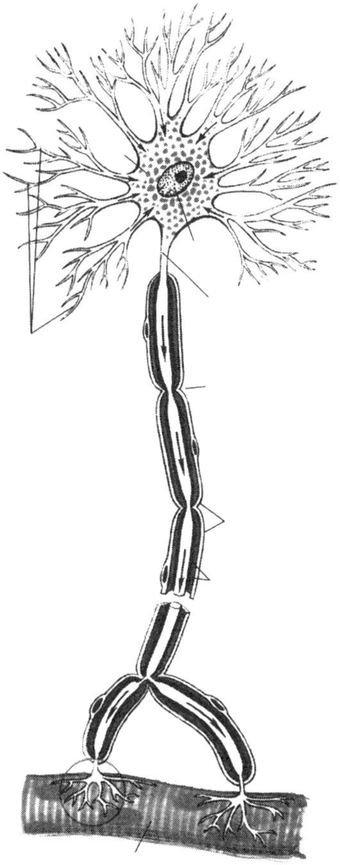

COMPETENCY EVALUATION CHECKLIST

Procedure 12-1 Assisting With a Lumbar Puncture

NAME ______________________ **DATE/TIME** ______________

EVALUATED __________ ______________________ **SCORE** ______________

Goal—To assist with a lumbar puncture.

Objectives/Conditions—When assigned to assist with a lumbar puncture, the student will obtain appropriate equipment and supplies, then the student will demonstrate how to correctly assist with this type of procedure.

Outcome—The student correctly assists with a lumbar puncture in accordance with the steps presented in the text.

Equipment and Supplies

On the sterile field

3–5 inch lumbar needle with a stylet (physician will specify gauge and length)
Gloves for the physician
Gauze sponges
Specimen tubes for transport
Spinal fluid manometer with a 3-way stopcock adapted (if CSF pressure is to be measured)
Fenestrated drape
Sterile drape
Antiseptic

On the side

Local anesthetic and syringe
Adhesive bandages
Sterile gloves (if not included on the field)
Examination gloves for the assistant
Skin preparation supplies
Blood pressure cuff (if Queckenstedt test is to be performed)
Completed lab slips for CSF

Steps	**Y**	**N**	**Number of Attempts**
1. Wash your hands.	☐	☐	______
2. Assemble the equipment. (Most offices stock the equipment in a purchased disposable tray or a site-prepared setup.)	☐	☐	______
3. Gather personal protective equipment (eg, gloves) as needed.	☐	☐	______
4. Identify the patient.	☐	☐	______
5. Check that the consent form is signed and posted on the chart.	☐	☐	______
6. Explain that the puncture will be made below the level of the spinal cord and should present no danger to the patient. Warn the patient not to move during the procedure. Tell the patient that the area will be numbed but that pressure may still be felt after the local anesthetic is administered.	☐	☐	______
7. Have the patient void.	☐	☐	______
8. Direct the patient to disrobe and put on a gown with the opening in the back.	☐	☐	______
9. Determine and record the vital signs.	☐	☐	______

Steps (Continued)	Y	N	Number of Attempts
10. When the physician is ready, open the field (follow the steps described in Procedure 6-1, Opening Sterile Surgical Packs, in Chap. 6, Assisting With Minor Office Surgery), and assist with the initial preparations.	☐	☐	______
11. Prepare the skin if this is not done as part of the sterile preparation. Many physicians prefer to prepare the skin using a sterile forceps after gloving. If this is the preferred procedure, you may be required to add sterile solutions to the field (follow the steps in Procedure 6-3, Adding Sterile Solution to a Sterile Field in Chap. 6, Assisting With Minor Office Surgery).	☐	☐	______
12. Assist as needed with administration of the anesthetic.	☐	☐	______
13. Assist the patient into the appropriate position.	☐	☐	______
	☐	☐	______
a. *Side-lying position*	☐	☐	______
b. *Forward-leaning, supported position*	☐	☐	______
14. Throughout the procedure, observe the patient closely for signs such as dyspnea or cyanosis. Monitor the pulse at intervals.	☐	☐	______
15. When the physician has the needle securely in place, help the patient to straighten slightly to ease tension and to allow a more normal CSF flow. The physician may now use the stopcock and spinal fluid manometer to determine the intracranial pressure.	☐	☐	______
16. If specimens are to be taken, assist as follows:	☐	☐	______
a. Put on gloves to receive the potentially hazardous body fluid.	☐	☐	______
b. As you receive the tubes, label them in sequence and with the patient's identification.	☐	☐	______
c. Place the tubes in biohazard specimen bags.	☐	☐	______
Note: The first tube may be more likely to contain contaminants.	☐	☐	______
17. If the Queckenstedt test is to be performed, assist as follows:	☐	☐	______
Method one:			
• Press the veins of the patient's neck with your hands, first the right, then the left, then both sides, each for 10 seconds, while the physician measures the pressure with the stopcock and manometer.	☐	☐	______
Method two:			
• Before gloving for the procedure, the physician will place a blood pressure cuff around the patient's neck. According to the physician's instructions, inflate the cuff to 22 mm Hg for 10 seconds while the physician measures the pressure with the manometer.	☐	☐	______

Steps (Continued)	Y	N	Number of Attempts
18. At the completion of the procedure, perform these measures:			
a. Cover the site with an adhesive bandage.	☐	☐	______
b. Assist the patient to a supine position.	☐	☐	______
c. Record the patient's vital signs. Note mental alertness, any leakage at the site, nausea, and vomiting. Assess lower limb mobility. *Note:* The physician will determine when the patient is ready to leave the examining room and the office.	☐	☐	______
19. Route the specimens as required.	☐	☐	______
20. Clean the room and care for or dispose of the equipment as needed. Wash your hands.	☐	☐	______

☐ **Pass** ☐ **Fail**

Comments

____

____

____

____

13

Assisting With Diagnostic and Therapeutic Procedures Associated With the Sensory System

COMPETENCY PRACTICE

Vocabulary Assessment

Matching

Match the definition in Part 1 with the correct term in Part 2.

PART 1

1. pressure within the eyeball
2. farsightedness
3. nearsightedness
4. unfocused refraction of light rays on the retina
5. vision changes resulting from age
6. pathological changes in the retina
7. extraneous noise in one or both ears

PART 2

a. _____ retinal degeneration
b. _____ presbyopia
c. _____ tinnitus
d. _____ intraocular pressure
e. _____ hyperopia
f. _____ myopia
g. _____ astigmatism

Definitions

Define the following terms.

1. adnexa

____

____

____

2. cerumen

____

____

____

3. decibel

____

____

____

4. optician

5. optometrist

6. refraction

7. tactile

Critical Thinking

1. What are the symptoms of otitis media in children? Specifically, what are the symptoms that would necessitate an appointment with a physician and a course of treatment?

2. What is strabismus? What is exotropic strabismus? What is the treatment?

Case Studies

1. Allan Smith is 17 years old. He swims competitively for his high school. He arrives at his physician's office complaining of left ear pain for 2 days, as well as jaw pain. After examination, Dr. Jones tells Allan that he has "swimmers ear." He prescribes amoxicillin 250 mg four times a day for 10 days. He also advises Allan to wear ear plugs when he swims. What is swimmers ear? What causes it?

2. Allison is 5 years old and is scheduled for a physical examination in preparation for attending kindergarten in the fall. As part of the examination, her far vision will be tested. What chart will be used and what are some of the considerations the medical assistant should be aware of before performing the examination?

CHARTING EXERCISE

With regard to Case Study #1, write a narrative chart note describing Allan's history, diagnosis, and treatment.

Document on the Patient's Chart:

- Date and time
- Notification of physician
- Patient complaints/concerns
- Patient education
- Your signature

Date/Time	Conditions/Lab Results Patient Communication

Basic Writing Activities

Skill Drills

1. Identify the three layers of the eye and describe their functions.

____

____

____

2. Identify the two types of eye musculature and their functions.

____

____

____

3. Identify the two tests used for far and near vision testing.
   a. Far vision

   ____

   ____

   ____

   b. Near vision

   ____

   ____

   ____

4. List six causes of hearing loss.

____

____

____

Fill-in-the-Blanks

1. A staphylococcal infection of the eyelid, commonly called a sty, is a _______________.
2. Corneal ulcers may be caused by:
   a. _______________
   b. _______________
   c. _______________
   d. _______________
   e. _______________
   f. _______________
   g. _______________
3. The _______________ or _______________ is also known as the _______________ ear.
4. Meniere's disease causes loss of _______________ and upsets the body's ability to maintain _______________.
5. Otosclerosis affects all of the ossicles, but most particularly the _______________ bone.

Innovative Activities

Labeling

Identify the organs of taste and smell.

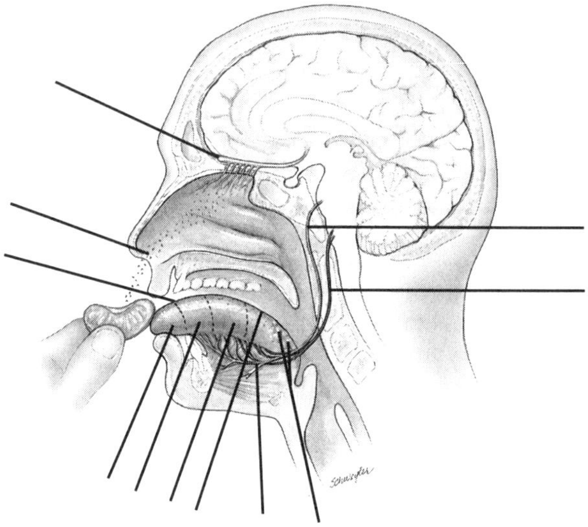

COMPETENCY EVALUATION CHECKLIST

Procedure 13-1 Preparing the Diagnostic Set

NAME ______________________ **DATE/TIME** ______________

EVALUATED ______________________ **SCORE** ______________

Goal—To prepare the diagnostic set.
Objectives/Conditions—When given equipment and supplies listed in the text, the student will prepare the diagnostic set.
Outcome—The student will prepare the diagnostic set in accordance with the steps in the text.

Equipment and Supplies

An operative otoscope, ophthalmoscope, and tongue blade holder (optional)
Power source, such as an electrical charger or fresh battery

Steps	Y	N	Number of Attempts
1. Wash your hands.	☐	☐	________
2. Assemble the equipment.	☐	☐	________
3. Check to determine that the lights in the instrument are functioning by illuminating them.	☐	☐	________
4. Place and remove the otoscope, ophthalmoscope, and illuminated tongue blade holder, if used, to check the readiness of each. Press firmly and twist to place or remove the head. The small red button at the connection is held down as the rim is rotated to keep the light on. Reverse the procedure to turn it off.	☐	☐	________
5. Place tongue blades and disposable ear specula on a covered tray for the physician's use.	☐	☐	________
6. Have extra light bulbs available for replacement during the examination if needed.	☐	☐	________

☐ **Pass** ☐ **Fail**

Comments

____

____

____

____

Procedure 13-2 Measuring Distance Visual Acuity

NAME ______________________ **DATE/TIME** ______________

EVALUATED ______________________ **SCORE** ______________

Goal—To measure distance visual acuity.
Objectives/Conditions—When given equipment and supplies listed in the text, the student will measure distance visual acuity.
Outcome—The student will accurately measure distance visual acuity in accordance with steps in the text.

Equipment and Supplies

Eye chart   Paper cup or eye paddle

Steps	Y	N	Number of Attempts
1. Wash your hands.	☐	☐	______
2. Prepare the examination room. Make sure the area is well lighted. A distance marker should be measured 20 feet from the chart; the chart must be at eye level.	☐	☐	______
3. Greet and identify the patient. Explain the procedure.	☐	☐	______
4. Position the patient in a standing or sitting position at the 20 foot marker.	☐	☐	______
5. Ask if the patient wears glasses or contact lenses. Mark the record accordingly.	☐	☐	______
6. Have the patient cover the left eye with the eye paddle. Instruct the patient to keep both eyes open.	☐	☐	______
7. Stand beside the chart and point to each row as the patient reads aloud the indicated lines, starting with the 20/200 line.	☐	☐	______
8. Record the smallest line the patient can read error free and note as OD (ocularis dexter). The numbers are listed on the side of the chart. For instance, if the patient reads line five (or the line marked 40) with one error for the right eye, record as OD 20/40 –1. Your physician may prefer that only those lines read without error be counted as correct.	☐	☐	______
9. Repeat the procedure with the right eye covered and record, using OS (ocularis sinistra). If the patient squints or leans forward, record this observation on the patient record.	☐	☐	______
10. Wash your hands.	☐	☐	______

☐ Pass   ☐ Fail

Comments

____

____

____

____

Procedure 13-3 Measuring Near Visual Acuity

NAME ______________________ **DATE/TIME** ______________

EVALUATED ______________________ **SCORE** ______________

Goal—To measure near visual acuity.
Objectives/Conditions—When given equipment and supplies listed in the text, the student will measure near visual acuity.
Outcome—The student will accurately measure near visual acuity in accordance with steps in the text.

Equipment and Supplies

Jaeger near visual acuity testing card
paper cup or eye paddle

Steps	Y	N	Number of Attempts
1. Wash your hands.	☐	☐	______
2. Assemble the equipment.	☐	☐	______
3. Greet and identify the patient. Explain the procedure. Ask for and answer any questions.	☐	☐	______
4. Hold the card containing lines of text or pictures of Es to be evaluated about 14 to 16 inches from the patient's face at a comfortable reading level.	☐	☐	______
5. Start by covering the patient's left eye.	☐	☐	______
6. Record the last line read with no errors.	☐	☐	______
7. Repeat the procedure to test the left eye.	☐	☐	______

☐ Pass ☐ Fail

Comments

____

____

____

____

Procedure 13-4 Measuring Color Perception

NAME ______________________ **DATE/TIME** ______________

EVALUATED ______________________ **SCORE** ______________

Goal—To measure color perception.
Objectives/Conditions—When given equipment and supplies listed in the text, the student will measure color perception.
Outcome—The student will accurately measure color vision in accordance with steps in the text.

Equipment and Supplies

Ishihara color plates
Gloves

Steps	Y	N	Number of Attempts
1. Wash your hands and put on gloves.	☐	☐	______
2. Identify the patient, and explain the procedure by the first plate. Hold the plate about 30 inches from the patient.	☐	☐	______
3. Ensure that the patient is in a comfortable sitting position in a quiet, well lighted room. Indirect sunlight gives the best illumination. (Sunlight should not shine against the plates; the colors fade with bright lights.)	☐	☐	______
4. Be aware that patients who wear glasses or contact lenses may keep them on.	☐	☐	______
5. Follow directions on the chart with the right eye, then the left eye.	☐	☐	______
6. Record the results of the test by noting what the patient reports as being seen on each plate, using the plate number and the answer given by the patient. If the patient cannot distinguish the pattern, record as Plate #3 = X. It is not necessary to record those read correctly. Record any squinting or tearing or any hesitation or guesses indicating that the patient was not sure of what was being perceived.	☐	☐	______
7. Store the book in a closed, protected area in its protective jacket to protect the integrity of the colors.	☐	☐	______

☐ Pass ☐ Fail

Comments

____
____
____
____

Procedure 13-5 Instilling Eye Medications

NAME ______________________ **DATE/TIME** ______________

EVALUATED ______________________ **SCORE** ______________

Goal—To instill eye medication.
Objectives/Conditions—When given equipment and supplies listed in the text, the student will instill eye medications.
Outcome—The student will instill eye medication in accordance with steps in the text.

Equipment and Supplies

Physician's order
Medication
Sterile gauze
Tissues

Steps	Y	N	Number of Attempts
1. Wash your hands and put on gloves.	☐	☐	______
2. Obtain the physician's order, the correct medication (check the label three times as directed in Chap. 8, Preparing and Administering Medications), and all needed supplies.	☐	☐	______
3. Greet and identify the patient. Explain the procedure. Ask the patient about allergies not recorded in the chart.	☐	☐	______
4. Position the patient comfortably.	☐	☐	______
5. Pull down the lower eyelid with sterile gauze and have the patient look upward.	☐	☐	______
6. Instill the medication.	☐	☐	______
a. *Ointment:* Discard the first bead of ointment. Place a thin line of ointment across the inside of the lower eyelid, moving from the inner canthus outward. Release the line of ointment by twisting slightly. Do not touch the tube to the eye.	☐	☐	______
b. *Drops:* Hold the dropper close to the conjunctival sac (about 1/2 inch away), but do not touch the patient. Release the proper number of drops into the sac. Discard any medication left in the dropper.	☐	☐	______
7. Have the patient gently close the eyelid and roll the eye to disperse the medication.	☐	☐	______
8. Wipe away any excess medication with the tissue. Instruct the patient to apply light pressure on the puncta for several minutes.	☐	☐	______
9. Properly care for or dispose of equipment and supplies. Clean the work area. Wash your hands.	☐	☐	______

☐ **Pass** ☐ **Fail**

Comments

____

____

____

____

Procedure 13-6 Irrigating the Eye

NAME ______________________ **DATE/TIME** ______________

EVALUATED ______________________ **SCORE** ______________

Goal—To irrigate the eye.

Objectives/Conditions—When given equipment and supplies listed in the text, the student will irrigate the eye.

Outcome—The student will irrigate the eye in accordance with steps in the text.

Equipment and Supplies

Small sterile basin
Towels
Emesis basin
Sterile irrigating solution at about 100 degrees F
Sterile bulb syringe
Tissues

Steps	Y	N	Number of Attempts
1. Wash your hands.	☐	☐	______
2. Assemble the equipment and supplies. Check the solution label three times as recommended for medication administration. Make sure the preparation is for ophthalmic purposes. *Note:* If both eyes are to be treated, use separate equipment for each to avoid cross-contamination.	☐	☐	______
3. Greet and identify the patient. Explain the procedure.	☐	☐	______
4. Position the patient comfortably, either sitting with head tilted with the affected eye downward or lying with the affected eye downward.	☐	☐	______
5. Drape the patient with a protective barrier to avoid wetting the clothing.	☐	☐	______
6. Have the patient hold the emesis basin against the upper cheek near the eye with the towel under the basin. Glove now. With clean gauze, wipe from the inner canthus outward to remove debris from the lashes.	☐	☐	______
7. Separate the lids with the thumb and forefinger of the nondominant hand. The dominant hand holding the syringe with solution may be lightly supported on the bridge of the patient's nose parallel to the eye to steady the hand.	☐	☐	______
8. Gently irrigate from the inner to the outer canthus, holding the syringe 1 inch above the eye. Use gentle pressure and do not touch the eye. The physician will order the period of time required for the irrigation.	☐	☐	______

Steps (Continued)	Y	N	Number of Attempts
9. Use tissue to wipe away any excess solution from the patient's face.	☐	☐	______
10. Properly dispose of equipment or sanitize as recommended and remove the gloves. Wash your hands.	☐	☐	______

☐ Pass ☐ Fail

Comments

______

______

______

______

Procedure 13-7 Assisting With Corneal Lavage

NAME ______________________ **DATE/TIME** ____________

EVALUATED ______ ______________________ **SCORE** ____________

Goal—To assist with corneal lavage.
Objectives/Conditions—When given equipment and supplies listed in the text, the student will assist with corneal lavage.
Outcome—The student will assist with corneal lavage in accordance with steps in the text.

Equipment and Supplies

Corneal lavage equipment (Morgan Lens, prescribed solution, fluid management system to receive outflow)
Topical ophthalmic solution
Sterile gloves

Steps	Y	N	Number of Attempts
1. Wash your hands.	☐	☐	______
2. Assemble equipment.	☐	☐	______
3. Greet and identify the patient. Explain the procedure. Ask about known allergies.	☐	☐	______
4. Help to position the patient, generally in a supine position with the affected eye downward.	☐	☐	______
5. Assist the physician as needed to administer the anesthetic drops.	☐	☐	______
a. Attach the irrigating solution to the lens apparatus.	☐	☐	______
b. Adjust the flow as the physician inserts the lens into the conjunctival sac.	☐	☐	______
6. Tape the tubing to the patient's forehead to prevent tension on the lens and accidental displacement. Attach the outflow device to collect the solution as it exits the eye.	☐	☐	______
7. As the physician removes the lens at the completion of the procedure, you may be required to stop the flow of solution after the removal.	☐	☐	______
8. Assist the patient to clean away excess fluid. Allow the patient to rest for a few moments before trying to stand.	☐	☐	______
9. Wash your hands. Care for or dispose of equipment as needed.	☐	☐	______

☐ **Pass** ☐ **Fail**

Comments

____

____

____

____

Procedure 13-8 Removing a Foreign Object From the Eye

NAME ______________________ **DATE/TIME** ______________

EVALUATED ______________________ **SCORE** ______________

Goal—To remove a foreign object from the eye.

Objectives/Conditions—When given equipment and supplies listed in the text, the student will remove a foreign object from the eye.

Outcome—The student will remove a foreign object from the eye in accordance with the steps in the text.

Equipment and Supplies

Sterile, cotton-tipped applicator
Sterile water or saline
Sterile medicine dropper or small bulb syringe
Tissues
Sterile gauze

Steps	Y	N	Number of Attempts
1. Wash your hands.	☐	☐	______
2. Assemble the equipment and supplies.	☐	☐	______
3. Greet and identify the patient. Explain the procedure.	☐	☐	______
4. Glove now. With the gauze against the cheek, pull down the lower eyelid and check for the object. If it is seen, moisten the applicator with the water or saline and gently try to remove the object.	☐	☐	______
5. If the object is not found on the lower lid, grasp the lashes of the upper lid and pull gently upward, checking for the upper surfaces of the eye for the object.	☐	☐	______
6. Perform an eye irrigation if necessary, following the steps in Procedure 13-6.	☐	☐	______
7. Wipe away an excess liquid with the tissue. Remove and dispose of the gloves.	☐	☐	______
8. Properly care for or dispose of equipment and supplies. Clean the work area. Wash your hands.	☐	☐	______

☐ Pass ☐ Fail

Comments

____

____

____

____

Procedure 13-9 Perform Audiometry

NAME ______________________ **DATE/TIME** ______________

EVALUATED ______________________ **SCORE** ______________

Goal—To perform audiometry.
Objectives/Conditions—When given equipment and supplies listed in the text, the student will perform audiometry.
Outcome—The student will perform audiometry in accordance with the steps in the text.

Equipment and Supplies

Audiometer
Disposable scope cover

Steps	Y	N	Number of Attempts
1. Wash your hands.	☐	☐	______
2. Assemble the equipment.	☐	☐	______
3. Greet and identify the patient. Escort the patient to a quiet room free of distractions. Explain the procedure.	☐	☐	______
4. Cover the probe with the disposable scope cover.	☐	☐	______
5. Position the auricle and canal by gently pulling up and back on the pinna for adults and down and back for small children to straighten the canal.	☐	☐	______
6. Insert the probe into the patient's ear. Visualize the tympanic membrane. Turn on the machine.	☐	☐	______
7. Practice with the patient using the pretone.	☐	☐	______
8. Select the testing level for the patient. Depress the "start" button. Observe the tone indicators and the patient's response.	☐	☐	______
9. Screen the opposite ear.	☐	☐	______
10. If the patient fails to respond at any frequency, retest through the procedure.	☐	☐	______
11. Remove and dispose of the probe cover. Wash your hands. Care for the equipment, and return the instrument to its charging base.	☐	☐	______

☐ Pass ☐ Fail

Comments

____

____

____

____

Procedure 13-10 Irrigate the Ear

NAME ______________________ **DATE/TIME** ______________

EVALUATED ______________________ **SCORE** ______________

Goal—To irrigate the ear.
Objectives/Conditions—When given equipment and supplies listed in the text, the student will irrigate the ear.
Outcome—The student will irrigate the ear in accordance with the steps in the text.

Equipment and Supplies

Irrigation solution of the physician's choice at no more than 100 degrees F (about 37 degrees C)
Basin for solution
Ear irrigation syringe or irrigating device
Waterproof barrier
Otoscope
Emesis basin or ear basin for outflow
Unsterile gauze

Steps	Y	N	Number of Attempts
1. Wash your hands.	☐	☐	______
2. Assemble the equipment and supplies.	☐	☐	______
3. Greet and identify the patient. Explain the procedure.	☐	☐	______
4. Position the patient comfortably in an erect position.	☐	☐	______
5. View the affected ear with an otoscope to locate the problem.	☐	☐	______
Adults: Gently pull up and slightly back to straighten the auditory canal.	☐	☐	______
Children: Gently pull slightly down and back to straighten the auditory canal.	☐	☐	______
Note: Do not irrigate if the tympanic membrane appears to be perforated without checking with the physician; solution may be forced into the middle ear through the perforation. Remove any obvious debris at the entrance of the canal before beginning the irrigation.	☐	☐	______
6. Drape the patient with a waterproof barrier.	☐	☐	______
7. Tilt the patient's head toward the affected side.	☐	☐	______
8. Place the drainage basin beneath the affected ear.	☐	☐	______
9. Fill the syringe, or turn on the irrigating device.	☐	☐	______
10. Gently position the auricle as described above with the nondominant hand.	☐	☐	______
11. With the dominant hand, place the tip of the syringe into the auditory meatus, and direct the flow of solution gently upward toward the roof of the canal.	☐	☐	______
12. Continue irrigating for the prescribed period of time.	☐	☐	______

Steps (Continued)	Y	N	Number of Attempts
13. Dry the patient's external ear with gauze. Have the patient sit for awhile with the affected ear downward to drain the solution.	☐	☐	______
14. Inspect the ear with the otoscope to determine the results.	☐	☐	______
15. Properly care for or dispose of equipment and supplies. Clean the work area. Wash your hands.	☐	☐	______

☐ **Pass** ☐ **Fail**

Comments

____

____

____

____

Procedure 13-11 Instill Ear Medication

NAME ______________________ **DATE/TIME** ______________

EVALUATED ______________________ **SCORE** ______________

Goal—To instill ear medication.
Objectives/Conditions When given equipment and supplies listed in the text, the student will instill ear medication.
Outcome—The student will instill ear medication in accordance with the steps in the text.

Equipment and Supplies

Medication formulated for otic purposes, with dropper
Cotton balls

Steps	Y	N	Number of Attempts
1. Wash your hands.	☐	☐	______
2. Assemble the equipment.	☐	☐	______
3. Check the medication three times as specified for medication administration. It must specify otic preparation.	☐	☐	______
4. Greet and identify the patient. Explain the procedure.	☐	☐	______
5. Have the patient seated with the affected ear tilted upward.	☐	☐	______
6. Draw up the ordered amount of medication.	☐	☐	______
7. Position the auricle.	☐	☐	______
Adults: Pull the auricle slightly up and back to straighten the S-shaped canal.	☐	☐	______
Children: Pull the auricle slightly down and back to straighten the S-shaped canal.	☐	☐	______
8. Insert the tip of the dropper without touching the patient's skin, and let the medication flow along the side of the canal.	☐	☐	______
9. Have the patient sit or lie with the affected ear upward for a short while.	☐	☐	______
10. If the medication is to be retained, insert the cotton ball slightly into the external auditory meatus without force.	☐	☐	______
11. Properly care for or dispose of equipment and supplies. Clean the work area. Wash your hands.	☐	☐	______

☐ Pass ☐ Fail

Comments

____

____

____

____

Procedure 13-12 Instill Nasal Medication

NAME ______________________ **DATE/TIME** ______________

EVALUATED ______________________ **SCORE** ______________

Goal—To instill nasal medication.
Objectives/Conditions—When given equipment and supplies listed in the text, the student will instill nasal medication.
Outcome—The student will instill nasal medication in accordance with the steps in the text.

Equipment and Supplies

Medication (drops or spray)
Nonsterile tissues

Steps	Y	N	Number of Attempts
1. Wash your hands.	☐	☐	______
2. Assemble the equipment and supplies. Check the medication label three times.	☐	☐	______
3. Greet and identify the patient. Explain the procedure. Ask the patient about allergies not documented.	☐	☐	______
4. Position the patient in a comfortable recumbent position. Extend the patient's head beyond the edge of the examination table, or place a pillow under the patient's shoulders. Support the patient's neck to avoid strain as the head is tilted back.	☐	☐	______
5. Glove now. Administer the medication.	☐	☐	______
a. Administer nose drops by holding the dropper upright just above each nostril and dropping the medication one drop at a time without touching the nares. Keep the patient in the recumbent position for 5 minutes.	☐	☐	______
b. Administer nasal spray by having the patient sit. Place the tip of the dispenser at the nare opening without touching the patient's skin or nasal tissues, and spray as the patient takes a deep breath.	☐	☐	______
6. Wipe away any excess medication from the patient's skin with tissues.	☐	☐	______
7. Properly care for or dispose of equipment and supplies. Clean the work area. Remove gloves. Wash your hands.	☐	☐	______

☐ Pass ☐ Fail

Comments

____
____
____
____

14

Assisting With Diagnostic and Therapeutic Procedures Associated With the Endocrine System

COMPETENCY PRACTICE

Vocabulary Assessment

Matching

Match the hormone or chemical in Part 1 with the area of the body where it is produced in Part 2.

PART 1

1. oxytocin
2. prolactin
3. calcitonin
4. epinephrine
5. glucocorticoids

PART 2

a. _____ adrenal cortex

b. _____ adrenal medulla

c. _____ thyroid gland

d. _____ anterior lobe, pituitary gland

e. _____ posterior lobe, pituitary gland

Definitions

Define each of the following terms.

1. endemic

____

____

____

2. goiter

____

____

____

3. glycosuria

____

____

____

4. hyperplasia

____

____

____

5. myxedema

6. polydipsia

7. pruritus

8. tetany

Critical Thinking

1. Explain the relationship between iodine and the development of a simple goiter. Include the consequences of gland enlargement and describe treatment of the condition.

2. Epinephrine is secreted in response to need, as in the flight or fight syndrome. Describe the physical effects of epinephrine secretion.

Case Studies

1. Mrs. Walker is a 52-year-old patient who has just been diagnosed with diabetes mellitus type II. Dr. Abrams has prescribed an oral hypoglycemic medication and a well-balanced diet and has encouraged Mrs. Walker to exercise regularly. As Mrs. Walker leaves the office, she says "I am so glad that I do not have to take shots. My friend has diabetes too but she has to take shots twice a day. She has had to do this for 25 years. How is it that my friend has to take shots and I do not?" Explain the difference between type I and type II diabetes, and describe the difference in treatment.

2. Mr. Allison is a 34-year-old man with diabetes mellitus type I. He has successfully learned how to self-administer insulin. Mr. Allison has questions about the timing of his injections and meals. How can you educate Mr. Allison about the relationship between injections and meals?

CHARTING EXERCISE

Using the situation described in Case Study #2, write a narrative chart note describing your interaction with the patient.

Document on the Patient's Chart:

- Date and time
- Notification of physician
- Patient complaints/concerns
- Patient education
- Your signature

Date/Time	Conditions/Lab Results Patient Communication

Basic Writing Activities

Skill Drills

1. Explain the difference between diabetic coma and insulin shock.

____

____

____

2. What is diabetes insipidus and what are its symptoms?

____

____

____

3. Identify where in the body estrogen is produced and list six physical developments that are stimulated by estrogen.

____

____

____

4. Ketoacidosis is a serious problem for patients with IDDM. Explain why and describe the treatment.

____

____

____

Completion

Complete the following sentences.

1. The endocrine glands differ from the body's other glands (exocrine glands) because they are _______________.
2. The pituitary gland is also known as the _______________.
3. Iodine is essential to the production of the three thyroid hormones: thyroxine, triiodothyronine, and _______________.
4. The pineal body is situated in the _______________.
5. The gonads include the _______________ and _______________.

Innovative Activities

Create a new employee information sheet describing various laboratory tests and diagnostic procedures the physician may use to identify endocrine disorders.

15

Assisting With Diagnostic and Therapeutic Procedures Associated With the Cardiovascular System

COMPETENCY PRACTICE

Vocabulary Assessment

Matching

Match the definition in Part 1 with the correct term in Part 2.

PART 1

1. double sac of serous membrane enclosing the heart
2. middle layer of the heart muscle
3. innermost part of the heart wall
4. upper chamber of the heart
5. pumping chambers
6. supplies blood to the heart muscle
7. prevents backflow into the left lower chamber

PART 2

a. _____ atria

b. _____ pericardium

c. _____ aortic semilunar valve

d. _____ myocardium

e. _____ coronary arteries

f. _____ endocardium

g. _____ ventricles

Definitions

Define the following terms.

1. aneurysm

____

____

____

2. artifacts

____

____

____

3. depolarization

____

____

____

4. dextrocardia

5. leads

6. mediastinum

7. repolarization

Proper medical term

Area affected

Symptoms

Treatment

Critical Thinking

1. Mrs. Green is being seen in the office because of complaints of chronic fatigue, weight loss, and anorexia. After a physical examination and blood tests, Dr. Wright determines that Mrs. Green has pernicious anemia. What is pernicious anemia? What is the treatment?

2. Compare and contrast the signs and symptoms of a CVA and an MI.

   CVA

   MI

Case Studies

1. Dr. Tang has asked you to apply a Holter monitor to Mr. Andrews. Why would a Holter monitor be used instead of an ECG for diagnosis of cardiac problems? How may the record be programmed? What is the patient responsible for during this procedure?

2. Mrs. Burg is scheduled for a cardiac stress test and a thallium scan today. As you prepare for the tests, Mrs. Burg asks you what the difference is between them. She is very nervous regarding these tests. What is the difference between a stress test and a thallium scan? How can you reassure her?

Charting Exercise

With regard to Case Study #2, write a chart note documenting your interaction with Mrs. Burg.

Document on the Patient's Chart:
- Date and time
- Notification of physician
- Patient complaints/concerns
- Patient education
- Your signature

Date/Time	Conditions/Lab Results Patient Communication

Basic Writing Activities

Skill Drills

1. Trace the conduction of an electrical impulse through the heart.

___

2. List six possible symptoms of transient ischemic attacks (TIAs).

___

3. Identify the location of the following disorders.

   a. carditis

   ___

   b. pericarditis

   ___

   c. myocarditis

   ___

   d. endocarditis

   ___

4. List the six causes of aneurysms.

___

Fill-in-the-Blanks

1. Atherosclerotic coronary heart disease is also called ___.
2. Patients are diagnosed as hypertensive if their blood pressure is above ___.
3. Narrowing of the aortic valve leaflets is called ___.
4. The most common circulatory disease of the lower extremities is ___.
5. Stasis ulcers are diagnosed with the aid of ___.

Innovative Activities

Labeling

Identify the structures of the heart and great vessels.

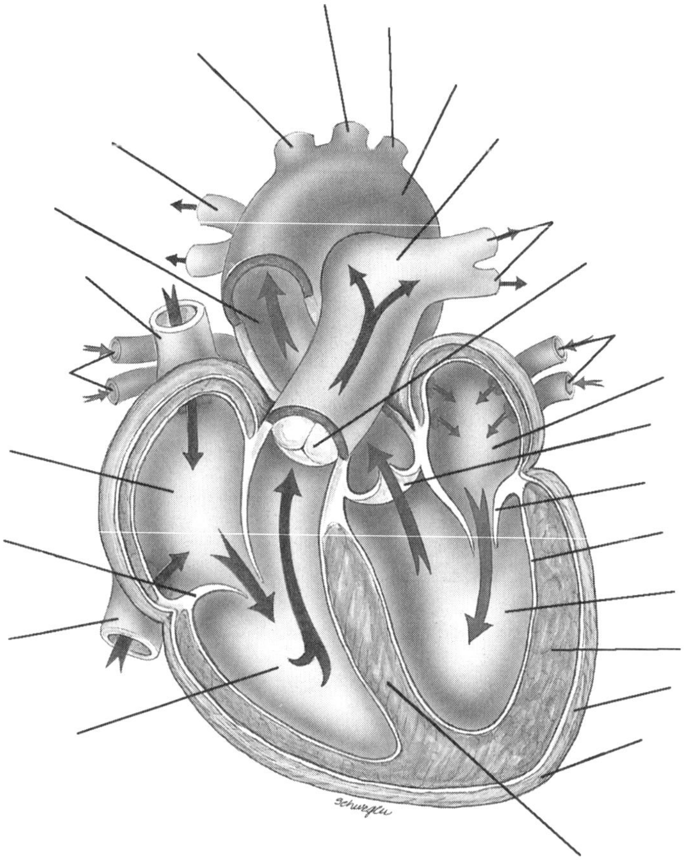

COMPETENCY EVALUATION CHECKLIST

Procedure 15-1 Perform a 12-Lead Electrocardiogram

NAME ______________________ **DATE/TIME** ______________

EVALUATED ______________________ **SCORE** ______________

Goal—To perform a 12-lead electrocardiogram.
Objectives/Conditions—When given equipment and supplies listed in the text, the student will perform a 12-lead electrocardiogram.
Outcome—The student will perform a 12-lead electrocardiogram in accordance with the steps in the text.

Equipment and Supplies

Equipment for measuring vital signs
ECG machine
ECG paper
Coupling gel or pads
Electrodes
Gown or cape
Razor (if necessary)
Comfortable table

Steps	Y	N	Number of Attempts
1. Wash your hands.	☐	☐	______
2. Assemble the equipment.	☐	☐	______
3. Greet and identify the patient. Explain the procedure, noting that the machine will pick up tremors or muscle movement and instructing the patient to lie still for the usually brief duration of the test. Ask for and answer any questions.	☐	☐	______
4. Before beginning the ECG, record the patient's data base: name, age, sex, height, weight, vital signs, symptoms, and medications. Note the time and date of the recording. *This information is needed for proper diagnosis.*	☐	☐	______
5. Note any preparation required for the test. Generally, no preparation is needed. However, the physician may request that the patient exercise for a prescribed time before the test to record changes brought about by physical stress. Also, skin preparation (eg, slight skin abrading or shaving) may be necessary for patients with extremely dry or oily skin, or for those with coarse arm or chest hair.	☐	☐	______
6. Instruct the patient to disrobe above the waist and provide a gown for privacy. Nylons or tights should be removed also.	☐	☐	______
7. Position the patient comfortably in a supine position with pillows as needed for comfort. Drape for warmth and privacy.	☐	☐	______
8. Check the machine for safety of grounding. Position it with the power cord away from the patient. Turn the machine on to warm the stylus.	☐	☐	______

Steps (Continued)	Y	N	Number of Attempts
9. Apply the electrodes according to the manufacturer's directions.	☐	☐	______
For metal electrodes:			
a. Apply a small amount of gel evenly and equally to all electrodes, or use a pad impregnated with electrolyte gel.	☐	☐	______
b. Rub the gel into the skin using the side of the electrode to redden the skin slightly for increased conduction.	☐	☐	______
c. Apply rubber straps to the prongs of the metal electrodes and attach snugly to the limbs.	☐	☐	______
For disposable electrodes: Be aware that disposable electrodes have electrolyte gel already applied equally and adequately. Place the electrodes on the skin (*Note:* Disposable electrodes adhere to the skin without straps.)	☐	☐	______
10. Be sure to place electrodes on the fleshy, muscular parts of the upper arms and lower legs. The attachments will point to the hands and feet of the patient.	☐	☐	______
11. If using Welch electrode cups for the chest leads, apply a small amount of electrolyte gel, compress the bulb to create a suction, press it against the patient's chest at first position, V_1, and release the bulb. Some chest leads may be attached with a rubber strap around the patient's chest, and others may be weighted with a metal strip.	☐	☐	______
12. Connect the leads securely. They will be coded RA, LA, LL, RL, and C-V. Some are color coded. Untangle the leads before applying to decrease electrical artifacts. Be sure that each lead lies unencumbered along the contours of the patient's body to decrease the incidence of artifacts. Double check the placement.	☐	☐	______
13. Plug in the cable and arrange it along the side of the patient on the table.	☐	☐	______
14. Center the stylus and press the standardization button (STD). Set on RUN 25. The mark should be 2×10 mm, or 2 small squares wide by 10 small squares high. Adjust appropriately within those parameters. Check at this time for artifacts.	☐	☐	______
15. Center the stylus on the paper and run 8–10 inches of leads I, II, III. If the R wave is too large for the reading, reduce the standardization to 1/2. If the reading is too small to be accurately read, increase the standardization $\times 2$. If you must move the stylus from the position of the standardization mark, make another mark for reference. If any of the leads are not properly attached, it will be apparent at this time.	☐	☐	______

Steps (Continued)	Y	N	Number of Attempts
16. If the leads were accurately placed and the stylus was appropriately centered for correct readings of leads I, II, III, then proceed manually to aVR, aVL, and aVF, if the machine does not progress automatically. Check the standardization each time a progression is made.	☐	☐	______
17. Switch to V_1 through V_6 for 5–6 inches of paper. If the instrument is not automatic, you will need to mark each lead as it is run (see Table 15-3 for standard marks).	☐	☐	______
18. If the machine does not progress automatically, and chest leads must be manually moved to the next position, turn off the machine before disconnecting the leads and restandardize each time. *Note:* If disposable electrode patches are used or if a myocardial infarction is suspected, the physician may want to check the reading before the electrodes are removed to avoid removing them and then replacing them for a repeat ECG run.	☐	☐	______
19. Turn off and unplug the machine at the completion of the reading.	☐	☐	______
20. Remove the electrodes and clean the patient's skin. Assist the patient from the table and help with dressing, as needed.	☐	☐	______
21. Carefully roll the ECG strip. Do not use clips to secure the roll.	☐	☐	______
22. Store the equipment by carefully coiling the leads. Clean the electrodes with kitchen cleanser if reusable.	☐	☐	______

☐ **Pass** ☐ **Fail**

Comments

____

____

____

____

Procedure 15-2 Mount an Electrocardiogram

NAME ______________________ **DATE/TIME** ______________

EVALUATED ______________________ **SCORE** ______________

Goal—To mount an electrocardiogram.
Objectives/Conditions—When given equipment and supplies listed in the text, the student will mount an electrocardiogram.
Outcome—The student will mount an electrocardiogram in accordance with the steps in the text.

Equipment and Supplies

Physician-preferred mounting device
Clean, flat surface
Scissors

Steps	Y	N	Number of Attempts
1. Label the mounting paper with the patient's data.	☐	☐	______
2. Unroll the strip on a clean, flat surface, and identify the area of lead I with the standardization mark. Cut this strip with scissors to the length preferred by the physician.	☐	☐	______
3. If the mounting device has protective sleeves, carefully open the sleeve as far as possible and insert the strip. If the mounting papers have adhesive strips and clear plastic covers, use care to prevent marring the surface of the strip.	☐	☐	______
4. Repeat the procedure until all of the leads are in their proper places on the chart.	☐	☐	______
5. File the report in the area the physician has designated for reports pending review.	☐	☐	______

☐ Pass ☐ Fail

Comments

____

____

____

____

Procedure 15-3 Apply a Holter Monitor for a 24-Hour Test

NAME ______________________ **DATE/TIME** ______________

EVALUATED ______________________ **SCORE** ______________

Goal—To apply a Holter monitor for a 24-hour test.

Objectives/Conditions—When given equipment and supplies listed in the text, the student will apply a Holter monitor for a 24-hour test.

Outcome—The student will apply a Holter monitor for a 24-hour test in accordance with the steps in the text.

Equipment and Supplies

Monitor
Fresh batteries
Roll of blank tape
Carrying case with strap
Electrodes
Skin swabs
Gauze
Razor (as needed)
Patient diary
Gloves, if skin must be shaved

Steps	Y	N	Number of Attempts
1. Assemble the equipment.	☐	☐	______
2. Greet and identify the patient. Explain the procedure. Remind the patient that it is important to carry out all normal activities for the duration of the test.	☐	☐	______
3. Explain the purpose for the incident diary, emphasizing the need for the patient to carry it at all times during the test.	☐	☐	______
4. Prepare the patient's skin for electrode attachment. Provide privacy and have the patient sit. Expose the chest, then shave the areas of attachment as needed. Glove, if shaving is required. Clean with the approved de-fatting agent to remove skin oils. Abrade the area with the gauze.	☐	☐	______
5. Apply the special Holter electrodes at the specified sites:			
a. The right manubrium border	☐	☐	______
b. The left manubrium border	☐	☐	______
c. The right sternal border at the fifth rib level	☐	☐	______
d. The fifth rib at the anterior axillary line	☐	☐	______
e. The right lower rib cage over the cartilage as a ground lead. To do this, expose the adhesive backing of the electrodes and follow manufacturer's instructions to attach firmly. Check for security of attachment.	☐	☐	______
Electrodes may also be placed at the left manubrium border at the level of the second rib and at the left sternal border at the fifth intercostal space.	☐	☐	______

Steps (Continued)	**Y**	**N**	**Number of Attempts**
6. Position electrode connectors downward toward the patient's feet. Attach the leads and secure with adhesive tape.	☐	☐	______
7. Connect the cable and run a baseline ECG by hooking the Holter to the ECG with the cable hookup.	☐	☐	______
8. Assist the patient to redress carefully with the cable extending through the garment opening. Clothing that buttons down the front is more convenient.	☐	☐	______
9. Plug the cable into the recorder and mark the diary. If needed, explain the purpose of the diary to the patient again. Give instructions for a return appointment to evaluate the recording and the diary.	☐	☐	______

☐ **Pass** ☐ **Fail**

Comments

____

____

____

____

16

Assisting With Diagnostic and Therapeutic Procedures Associated With the Immune System

COMPETENCY PRACTICE

Vocabulary Assessment

Matching

Match the definition in Part I with the correct term in Part 2.

PART I

1. produced in response to foreign antigens
2. chemical markers that identify cells
3. produced in response to injured cells
4. become mature antigen-specific cells in the spleen and lymph nodes
5. develop into mature differentiated lymphocytes
6. antibodies made by plasma
7. produced by cells infected by virus

PART 2

a. _____ interferon

b. _____ antibodies

c. _____ T-cells

d. _____ antihistamine

e. _____ B-cells

f. _____ antigen

g. _____ immune globulins

Word Scramble

Unscramble the following medical terms.

1. cavince

____

2. trite

____

3. gramapehoc

____

4. typehogac

____

5. xitood

____

Critical Thinking

1. Explain the difference between passive acquired natural immunity and passive acquired artificial immunity.

____

____

____

2. The spleen has several functions. List four.

____

____

____

Case Studies

1. Mr. Jones has been diagnosed with HIV. He will be returning to the office on a monthly basis to monitor his CD4 count. As you prepare to draw the blood for this test, Mr. Jones asks you to tell him again what the test is and what the results will mean for the physician's treatment plan. What can you tell Mr. Jones about a CD4 count and how will the results of this test affect his treatment?

____

____

____

2. Miss Adams is concerned about exposure to HIV. She has requested that Dr. Smith perform an HIV test. Miss Adams is very nervous about receiving the results of the test and wants to know how accurate the testing is. She specifically wants to know the name of the tests. How can you educate Miss Adams about the transmission of HIV? Explain the different tests and how they are used.

____

____

____

CHARTING EXERCISE

Using the situation in Case Study #1, write a narrative chart note describing your interaction with the patient, including the blood draw.

Document on the Patient's Chart:

- Date and time
- Notification of physician
- Patient complaints/concerns
- Patient education
- Your signature

Date/Time	Conditions/Lab Results Patient Communication

Basic Writing Activities

Skill Drills

1. List four disorders of the lymphatic and immune system.

____

____

____

2. Define HIV and AIDS.

____

____

____

3. Describe the four stages in the progression of HIV infection to AIDS.

____

____

____

4. List four methods of transmission of HIV and AIDS.

____

____

____

Fill-in-the-Blanks

1. Clear, watery fluid filtered from the blood in the capillaries is called ____________________.
2. Collections of stationary lymphatic tissue are called ____________________ and ____________________.
3. Lymph nodules of the pharynx are called ____________________.
4. The ____________________ contains lymphoid tissue designed to filter blood.
5. ____________________ is an inflammation of the lymphatic vessels.

Innovative Activities

Labeling

Label the Lymphatic System figure.

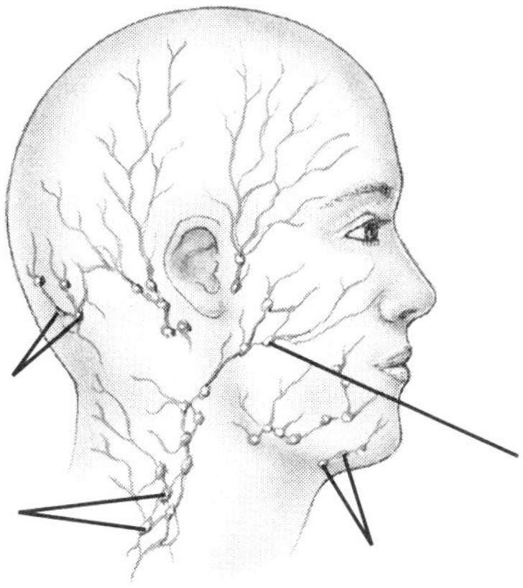

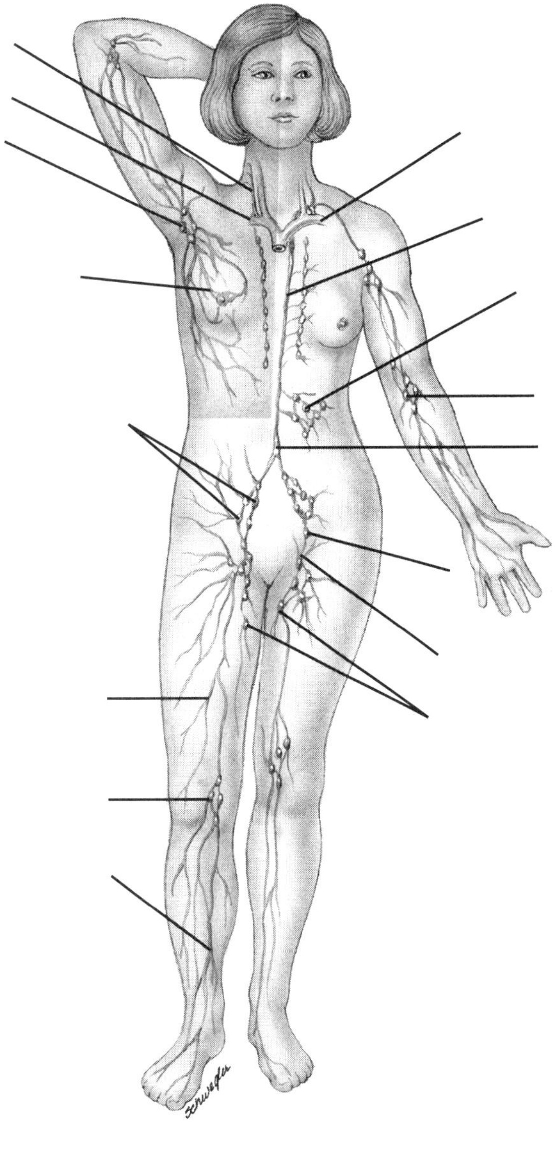

17

Assisting With Diagnostic and Therapeutic Procedures Associated With the Respiratory System

COMPETENCY PRACTICE

Vocabulary Assessment

Matching

Match the definition in Part 1 with the correct term in Part 2.

PART 1

1. bony projections of the nasal cavity walls
2. hollow cavities in the bones around the nose
3. common passageway of food, water, and air
4. connects the nasopharynx with the middle ear
5. pharyngeal tonsils
6. lymphoid tissue designed to prevent infection from spreading to the lower respiratory tract
7. "voice box"

PART 2

a. _____ eustachian tubes

b. _____ adenoids

c. _____ turbinates

d. _____ larynx

e. _____ tonsils

f. _____ paranasal cavities

g. _____ pharynx

Word Scramble

Unscramble the following letters to form a medical term.

1. ypaends

____

2. iicla

____

3. ssnoti

____

4. raacni

____

5. ulepar

____

6. gpietstioi

____

Critical Thinking

1. Why is it better to inhale through the nose rather than the mouth? Describe the structure and function of the nose to support your answer.

2. While COPD (chronic obstructive pulmonary disease) is not curable, the progress of the disease and the quality of life for patients can be improved in several ways. Discuss.

Case Studies

1. Dennis, 10 years of age, has asthma. The pediatrician has completed his examination and wants Dennis to use a peak flow meter as part of his treatment plan. While you are arranging a return appointment for Dennis, his mother asks you to explain the peak flow meter again so that she can be sure to help Dennis use it. What can you tell Dennis's mother about the purpose of the flow meter?

2. Jennifer, aged 15, is being seen for a fever to 102 (orally) for 2 days, a cough for 1 day, and sore throat for 3 days. Dr. Jones orders a throat culture. What is the purpose of a throat culture?

CHARTING EXERCISE

With regard to Case Study #2, write a chart note that documents Jennifer's reason for the office visit and any procedures that were performed.

Document on the Patient's Chart:

- Date and time
- Notification of physician
- Patient complaints/concerns
- Patient education
- Your signature

Date/Time	Conditions/Lab Results Patient Communication

Basic Writing Activities

Skill Drills

1. Explain the difference between external and internal respiration.

2. Identify five reasons for a tracheostomy.

3. Identify the three sets of tonsils and their location.

____

____

____

Fill-in-the-Blanks

1. Sputum specimens are generally ordered to be collected in the _________________.
2. The eustachian tube connects the nasopharynx to the _________________.
3. There are approximately _________________ million alveoli in the lungs of an adult.
4. Acute rhinitis, also called _________________, may be caused by _________________.
5. It is important that sputum be collected from the _________________.
6. The _________________ is the leaflike flap that prevents solids or liquids from entering the _________________.

Innovative Activities

Labeling

Identify the paranasal sinuses.

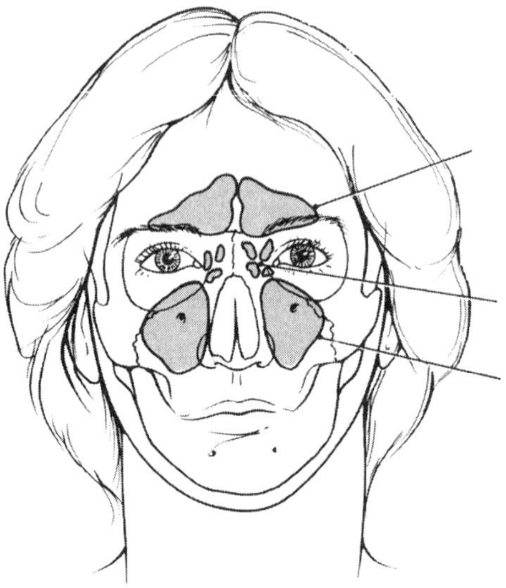

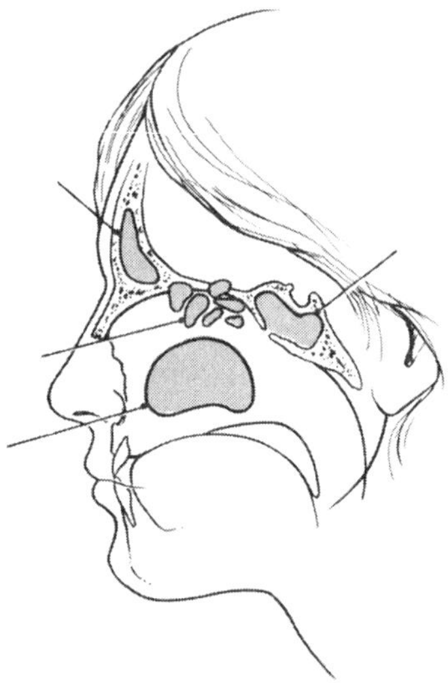

COMPETENCY EVALUATION CHECKLIST

Procedure 17-1 Collecting a Specimen for Throat Culture

NAME ______________________ **DATE/TIME** ______________

EVALUATED ______________________ **SCORE** ______________

Goal—To collect a specimen for throat culture.

Objectives/Conditions—When given equipment and supplies listed in the text, the student will collect a specimen for throat culture.

Outcome—The student will collect a specimen for throat culture in accordance with the steps in the text.

Equipment and Supplies

Tongue blade (depressor)
Sterile specimen container
Sterile swab (if one is not supplied with the specimen container)
Completed laboratory request slip

Steps	Y	N	Number of Attempts
1. Wash your hands.	☐	☐	______
2. Assemble the equipment and supplies.	☐	☐	______
3. Greet and identify the patient. Explain the procedure.	☐	☐	______
4. Have the patient sit with a light source directed at the throat.	☐	☐	______
5. Put on gloves and face mask or shield.	☐	☐	______
6. Carefully remove the sterile swab from the container.	☐	☐	______
7. Have the patient say "AHHH" as you press on the midpoint of the tongue with the tongue depressor.	☐	☐	______
8. Swab the areas of concern on the mucous membranes, especially the tonsillar area, the crypts, and the posterior pharynx. Turn the swab to expose all of its surfaces. Avoid touching areas other than those suspected of infection.	☐	☐	______
9. Maintain the tongue depressor position while withdrawing the swab.	☐	☐	______
10. Follow the instructions on the specimen container for transferring the swab. Some require that the wooden swab stick be broken after dropping into the culture; others may have a special swab that is contained within the cap and is secured when the container is sealed.	☐	☐	______

Steps (Continued)	Y	N	Number of Attempts
11. Properly dispose of the equipment and supplies. Remove gloves and wash your hands.	☐	☐	______
12. Route the specimen or store it appropriately until routing can be completed.	☐	☐	______

☐ **Pass** ☐ **Fail**

Comments

______

______

______

______

Procedure 17-2 Collecting a Sputum Specimen for Culture or Cytologic Examination

NAME ______________________ ____________ **DATE/TIME** ______________

EVALUATED ______________________________ **SCORE** ____________

Goal—To collect a sputum specimen for culture or cytologic examination.

Objectives/Conditions—When given equipment and supplies listed in the text, the student will collect a sputum specimen for culture or cytologic examination.

Outcome—The student will collect a specimen for culture or cytologic examination in accordance with the steps in the text.

Equipment and Supplies

Labeled sterile specimen container

Cover bag

Steps	Y	N	Number of Attempts
1. Wash your hands.	☐	☐	______
2. Assemble the equipment.	☐	☐	______
3. Greet and identify the patient. Explain the procedure.	☐	☐	______
4. Put on gloves and, if necessary, face shield and impervious gown (if you are assisting the patient with sputum collection).	☐	☐	______
5. Have the patient brush his or her teeth or rinse his or her mouth well.	☐	☐	______
6. Have the patient cough deeply, using the abdominal muscles and the accessory muscles to bring secretions from the lung fields and not just the upper airways.	☐	☐	______
7. Have the patient expectorate directly into the specimen container without touching the inside and without getting sputum on the sides of the container. About 5–10 mL is usually needed.	☐	☐	______
8. Handle the specimen observing Standard Precautions. Cap the container immediately, and drop it into the cover container.	☐	☐	______
9. Assist the patient to rinse his or her mouth after collecting the specimen.	☐	☐	______
10. Properly care for or dispose of equipment and supplies. Clean the work area. Remove gloves, gown, and face shield and wash your hands.	☐	☐	______
11. Process the specimen immediately, or within 2 hours, to avoid compromising the studies.	☐	☐	______

☐ Pass ☐ Fail

Comments

____

____

____

____

18

Assisting With Diagnostic and Therapeutic Procedures Associated With Gastrointestinal Disorders

COMPETENCY PRACTICE

Vocabulary Assessment

Matching

Match the definition in Part 1 with the correct term in Part 2.

PART 1

1. rhythmic wave action of the intestines
2. taste buds
3. teeth breaking food into manageable pieces
4. food lifted by the tongue and moved to the otopharynx
5. flow backward
6. stomach folds present when the stomach is empty
7. thick liquids in the stomach

PART 2

a. _____ mastication

b. _____ reflux

c. _____ rugae

d. _____ papillae lingua

e. _____ deglutition

f. _____ chyme

g. _____ peristalsis

Definitions

Define the following terms.

1. ascites

____

____

____

2. bolus

____

____

____

3. chyle

____

____

____

4. guaiac

____

____

____

5. melena

____

____

____

6. obstipation

____

____

____

Critical Thinking

Answer these questions on a separate sheet of paper.

1. Explain the action of anabolism and catabolism.
2. You are training a new employee in some basic procedures and tests that are commonly performed in the office. Today you will explain occult blood, disorders that may cause gastrointestinal bleeding, and screening methods used to detect the presence of blood in the stool. You will also explain the need to follow Universal Precautions. What information will you give the new employee?

Case Studies

1. Mr. Zamora, aged 50, is scheduled for a barium enema, which will be performed 3 days from today. He has an appointment today at 2:30 p.m. for a brief examination. You escort him to a room and obtain his vital signs (T 98.6, P 80, R 16, and BP 120/80). At the end of the exam, at 3:00 p.m., the physician asks you to give Mr. Zamora a bowel preparation brochure and to be sure that the patient understands what he needs to do before the bowel study. What information would you expect to be included in the brochure?

____

____

____

2. (Continued from Case Study #1.) Mr. Zamora goes home, but calls you at 5:15 p.m. and asks "why is a liquid diet without dairy products important the day before I have the barium enema? Wouldn't a light regular meal be fine?" How will you educate Mr. Zamora to the need to closely follow the bowel preparation directions?

____

____

____

CHARTING EXERCISE

Using the situations in Case Study #1 and #2, write narrative chart notes describing your interactions with the patient.

Document on the Patient's Chart:

- Date and time
- Notification of physician
- Patient complaints/concerns
- Patient education
- Your signature

Date/Time	Conditions/Lab Results Patient Communication

Basic Writing Activities

Skill Drills

1. List and describe the four main regions of the stomach.

____

____

____

2. Identify the six primary organs of the gastrointestinal system.

____

____

____

3. List the three accessory organs of the gastrointestinal system.

____

____

____

4. Identify six colon disorders.

____

____

____

Fill-in-the-Blanks

Complete the following sentences with the correct medical term.

1. Food is broken down into usable units by a process of physical and chemical changes called _____________________.
2. The most common disease of the mouth tissues is _____________________.
3. Inflammation of the gingiva is called _____________________.
4. A chronic inflammatory disease of the lining of the colon is _____________________.
5. Dilated veins in the rectum are called _____________________.

Innovative Activities

Labeling

Identify and label the diagrams.

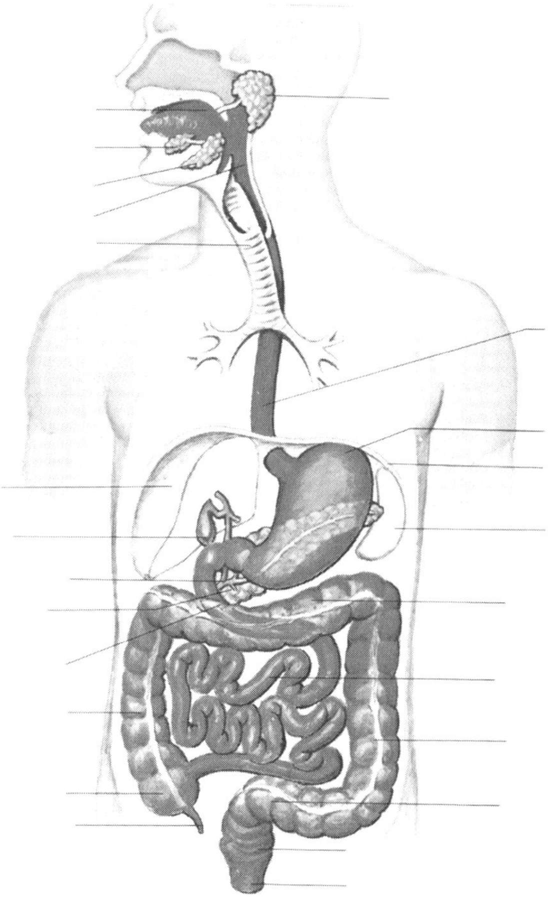

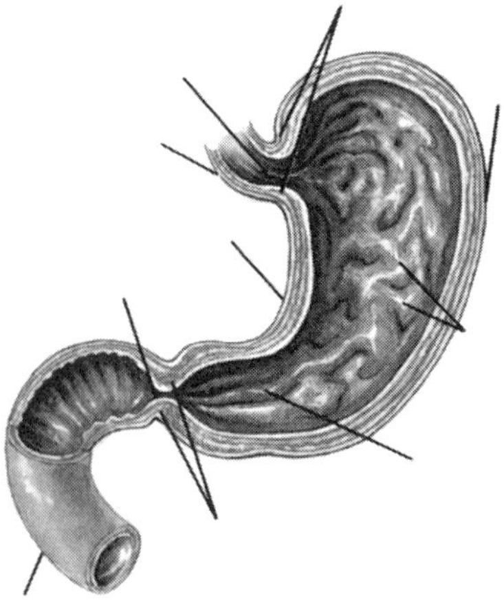

COMPETENCY EVALUATION CHECKLIST

Procedure 18-1 Preparing a Patient for Procedures Pertaining to the Colon

NAME ______________________ **DATE/TIME** ______________

EVALUATED ______________________ **SCORE** ________

Goal—To prepare a patient for a colon procedure.

Objectives/Conditions—When asked to prepare a patient for a colon procedure, the student will obtain appropriate equipment and supplies and correctly demonstrate how a patient is to be prepared.

Outcome—The preparation of a patient for procedures pertaining to the colon is performed in accordance with the steps presented in the text.

Equipment and Supplies

Appropriate instrument (flexible or rigid sigmoidoscope, anoscope, or proctoscope)
Water-soluble lubricant
Fenestrated drape or gown
Cotton swabs
Suction source (if not part of the scope)
Biopsy forceps
Specimen container with preservative
Completed laboratory requests
Personal wipes
Equipment for assessing vital signs

Steps	Y	N	Number of Attempts
1. Wash your hands.	☐	☐	______
2. Assemble the equipment.	☐	☐	______
3. Check the illumination of the light source. Turn off the power to avoid a buildup of heat.	☐	☐	______
4. Greet and identify the patient. Explain the procedure. The patient will feel pressure and may have the urge to defecate. Tell the patient that the pressure is from the instrument and that the feeling will ease. The patient also may experience gas pressure when air is insufflated. *Note:* Some patients are ordered a mild sedative before the procedure.	☐	☐	______
5. Instruct the patient to empty the bladder.	☐	☐	______
6. Assess the vital signs and record.	☐	☐	______
7. Have the patient undress from the waist down or undress completely and put on a gown.	☐	☐	______
8. Assist the patient onto the table. If the instrument of choice is an anoscope or a fiberoptic device, Sims' position or a left-lying position is most comfortable for the patient. If a rigid instrument is used, the patient will assume a knee-chest position or be placed on a proctologic table that supports the patient in a knee-chest position. *Note:* Do not ask the patient to assume the knee-chest position until the physician is ready to begin. The position is difficult to maintain, and the patient may become faint.	☐	☐	______

Steps (Continued)	Y	N	Number of Attempts
9. When the patient is in position, drape properly. A fenestrated drape usually is used.	☐	☐	______
10. Continually monitor the patient's response and offer reassurance during the examination. Instruct the patient to breathe slowly through pursed lips to aid in relaxation.	☐	☐	______
11. Assist the physician as needed with lubricants, instruments, power sources, swabs, biopsy equipment, and specimen containers. Glove before receiving biohazardous specimens.	☐	☐	______
12. Following the procedure, assist the patient into a comfortable position and allow a rest period. Offer personal cleaning wipes, and assist with cleaning as needed. Monitor the vital signs before allowing the patient to stand. Assist the patient from the table, and remain close at hand to avoid falls.	☐	☐	______
13. Have the patient dress.	☐	☐	______
14. Clean the room. Route the specimens to the proper laboratory. Clean or dispose of the supplies and equipment as appropriate, and wash your hands.	☐	☐	______

☐ Pass ☐ Fail

Comments

____

____

____

____

Procedure 18-2 Collecting a Stool Specimen

NAME ______________________ **DATE/TIME** ______________

EVALUATED ______________________ **SCORE** ______________

Goal—To collect a stool specimen.

Objectives/Conditions—When asked to collect a stool specimen, the student will obtain appropriate equipment and supplies and correctly demonstrate how to collect this type of specimen.

Outcome—A stool specimen is collected in accordance with the steps presented in the text.

Equipment and Supplies

Stool specimen container (usually waxed cardboard or plastic to avoid the transfer of pathogens through a moist container)
Wooden spatula or tongue blades
Bedpan with cover or toilet collection container (popularly called a "nun's cap" or "Mexican hat") with cover
Personal wipes for the patient

Steps	Y	N	Number of Attempts
1. Wash your hands.	☐	☐	________
2. Assemble the equipment.	☐	☐	________
3. Greet and identify the patient. Explain the procedure. Tell the patient to defecate in the bedpan or toilet collection container, not the toilet. The patient must void separately. Make sure the patient discards toilet tissue in the toilet and not in the bedpan or collection container.	☐	☐	________
4. Put on gloves, and obtain the bedpan or collection container from the patient. *Standard Precautions must be followed when handling stool.*	☐	☐	________
5. Using a tongue blade or wooden spatula, remove small portions of the stool from the bedpan or collection container. Take the specimens from the first and final portions of the stool. Transfer the stool to the specimen container. Do not allow feces to soil the outer surface of the specimen container.	☐	☐	________
6. Discard the supplies in biohazard containers, and flush the remaining stool.	☐	☐	________
7. Cap the specimen quickly and tightly. *This prevents loss of moisture, which may alter the results.*	☐	☐	________
8. Assist the patient with cleaning the rectal area. Have the patient wash his or her hands. *This provides comfort and promotes infection control.*	☐	☐	________
9. Clean, disinfect, and store or properly dispose of the bedpan or collection container. Remove gloves and wash hands after handling the specimen and supplies.	☐	☐	________

Steps (Continued)	Y	N	Number of Attempts
10. Label the specimen, and attach the laboratory requests.	☐	☐	________
11. Store the specimen as directed. Some require refrigeration, others are kept at room temperature, and some must be incubated. Check the office policy and procedure manual for recommendations for storage and routing of all specimens.	☐	☐	________

☐ Pass ☐ Fail

Comments

____

____

____

____

Procedure 18-3 Testing Stools for Occult Blood

NAME ______________________ **DATE/TIME** ______________

EVALUATED ______________________ **SCORE** ______________

Goal—To test stool for occult blood.

Objectives/Conditions—When asked to test a stool for occult blood, the student will obtain appropriate equipment and supplies and correctly demonstrate how to perform this type of test.

Outcome—A stool is tested for occult blood in accordance with the steps presented in the text.

Equipment and Supplies

Patient's labeled specimen pack
Developers or reagents

Steps	Y	N	Number of Attempts
1. Wash hands and put on gloves before receiving the specimen.	☐	☐	________
2. Identify the patient pack or the specimen from the physician. Depending on the testing method, the specimen may be tested as quickly as 3 to 5 minutes after collection or up to 14 days later if properly stored.	☐	☐	________
3. Open the window on the back of the pack, and apply the testing reagent or developer.	☐	☐	________
4. Read the color change in the specified time frame, usually 60 seconds.	☐	☐	________
5. Apply developers as directed onto the control monitor section of the pack. Wait the specified time.	☐	☐	________
6. Properly dispose of the pack, gloves, and supplies. Wash your hands.	☐	☐	________

☐ Pass ☐ Fail

Comments

____

____

____

____

19

Assisting With Diagnostic and Therapeutic Procedures Associated With the Urinary System

COMPETENCY PRACTICE

Vocabulary Assessment

Matching

Match the description in Part 1 with the correct term in Part 2.

PART 1

1. functional unit of kidney
2. twisted capillaries in Bowman's capsule
3. outer portion of kidney
4. inner portion of kidney
5. conical structures in renal medulla
6. funnel-shaped collecting basin
7. collecting structures
8. filtration takes place here
9. most dense portion of tubular system

PART 2

a. _____ calyces
b. _____ convoluted tubules
c. _____ glomerulus
d. _____ loop of Henle
e. _____ nephron
f. _____ renal cortex
g. _____ renal medulla
h. _____ renal pelvis
i. _____ renal pyramids

Definitions

Define the following terms.

1. angiotensin

____

____

2. erythropoietin

____

____

3. nitrogenous

____

____

4. pH

____

____

5. specific gravity

____

____

6. urea

____

____

7. uric acid

____

____

8. staghorn

____

____

Critical Thinking

1. Why is cystitis more common in women than in men? What advice could the medical assistant offer a female patient on prevention of this condition?

____

____

____

2. What are the advantages of peritoneal dialysis when compared to hemodialysis? Are certain patients not good candidates for peritoneal dialysis? Explain.

____

____

____

Case Studies

1. Mr. Lewis arrives at the office complaining of severe left flank pain for the past 3 hours. The medical assistant obtains a urine specimen and performs a urinalysis. Mr. Lewis is examined by Dr. English who reviews the lab reports and tells Mr. Lewis that he may have kidney stones. Dr. English orders an IV pyelogram. The results confirm the presence of stones and Mr. Lewis is scheduled for a lithotripsy the next day. Why are kidney stones so painful? What is lithotripsy?

____

____

____

2. Three weeks ago, Johnny, aged 6 years, had a severe streptococcal infection. On his visit today to Dr. Anderson's office, Johnny is diagnosed with glomerulonephritis. Johnny's mother is very concerned about the diagnosis and long-term complications. She wonders if she could have prevented this problem. Explain glomerulonephritis. Could Johnny's mother have prevented the problem? Why?

____

____

____

CHARTING EXERCISE

With regard to Case Study #1, write a chart note documenting Mr. Lewis's office visit.

Document on the Patient's Chart:

- Date and time
- Notification of physician
- Patient complaints/concerns
- Patient education
- Your signature

Date/Time	Conditions/Lab Results Patient Communication

Basic Writing Activities

Skill Drills

1. List the three waste products of metabolism excreted by the kidney.

___

___

___

2. List the six distinct organs of the urinary system and their function.

___

___

___

3. What is the difference between an intravenous pyelogram and a retrograde pyelogram?

___

___

___

4. Identify two common diagnostic procedures of the urinary system.

___

___

___

Completion

Complete the following sentences.

1. Red bone marrow will increase the production of red blood cells in response to the hormone ___.
2. The kidneys regulate blood level of calcium in conjunction with the ___.
3. There are ___ nephrons in each kidney.
4. ___ gallons of filtrate pass through the kidney in 24 hours.
5. The length of the male urethra is ___.
6. The length of the female urethra is ___.
7. The single most important diagnostic test for urinary system diseases is ___.

Innovative Activities

Labeling

Identify the parts of a nephron.

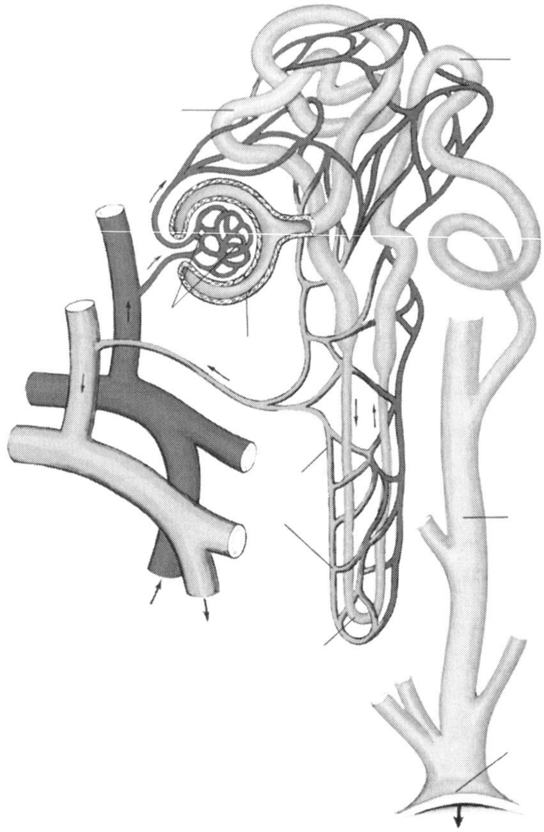

20

Assisting With Diagnostic and Therapeutic Procedures Associated With the Male Reproductive System

COMPETENCY PRACTICE

Vocabulary Assessment

Matching

Match the definition in Part 1 with the correct term in Part 2.

PART 1

1. sperm matures here
2. transports sperm
3. produces part of seminal fluid that contains fructose
4. produces additional seminal fluid
5. also called gametes
6. produces testosterone
7. male hormone

PART 2

a. _____ sperm/ovum
b. _____ testes
c. _____ testosterone
d. _____ epididymis
e. _____ seminal vesicles
f. _____ prostate
g. _____ vas deferens

Fill-in-the-Boxes

Fill-in the boxes with the correct term defined in the sentence.

1. tail of the sperm
☐☐☐☐☐☐☐☐☐
2. formation of sperm
☐☐☐☐☐☐☐☐☐☐☐☐☐☐☐
3. gland that encircles the urethra
☐☐☐☐☐☐☐☐
4. structure common to both urinary and reproductive systems
☐☐☐☐☐
5. glands that are comparable to the female's Bartholin glands
☐☐☐☐☐☐☐ ☐☐☐☐☐☐
6. term for undescended testes
☐☐☐☐☐☐☐☐☐☐☐☐☐☐

Critical Thinking

1. How would abstinence affect male fertility?

2. Would a vasectomy diminish the volume of ejaculate? Explain.

CASE STUDIES

1. On routine physical examination, Mr. Adams, aged 63, is found to have prostatic hypertrophy. Dr. Elder orders a PSA. Mr. Adams asks the medical assistant about the test when she gives him the laboratory slip. He wants to know why he has to have this test when Dr. Elder examined his prostate as part of the physical examination. What is a PSA test? What should the medical assistant tell Mr. Adams about PSA?

2. Mr. Jones, aged 24, has been diagnosed with herpes genitalis. Dr. Smith has obtained a urethral culture and given Mr. Jones a prescription for acyclovir. Dr. Smith asks you to send the specimen to the lab and give Mr. Jones his prescription. When scheduling a return appointment, Mr. Jones asks the medical assistant if acyclovir is a cure for the disease. Is it a cure for the disease? If not, what effect does it have on the disease?

CHARTING EXERCISE

With regard to Case Study #2, write a narrative chart note describing your interaction with the patient.

Document on the Patient's Chart:
- Date and time
- Notification of physician
- Patient complaints/concerns
- Patient education
- Your signature

Date/Time	Conditions/Lab Results Patient Communication

Basic Writing Activities

Skill Drills

1. List five characteristics of the male that are influenced by testosterone.

2. List four sexually transmitted diseases.

3. List four components of semen and their approximate percentages.

____

____

____

4. List five causes of male infertility

_______________ _______________

____

____

Fill-in-the-Blanks

1. The vas deferens, or _______________, is continuous with the epididymis.
2. The maturation process for sperm lasts _______________ days.
3. All men over age 40 should have a _______________ _______________ _______________ during yearly physical examinations.
4. A _______________, or collection of fluid within the scrotum and around the testes, may be the result of trauma or infection.
5. A _______________ testicle may result in sterility and can increase the risk of cancer in males.
6. A chancre is evident during the _______________ stage of syphilis.

Innovative Activities

Labeling

Identify the parts of a human spermatozoon.

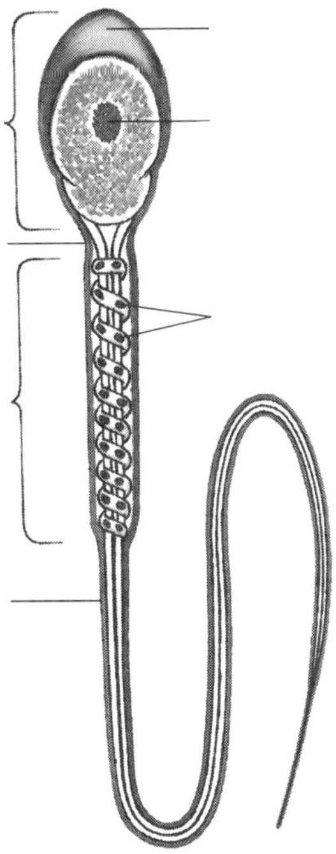

21

Assisting With Diagnostic and Therapeutic Procedures Associated With the Female Reproductive System

COMPETENCY PRACTICE

Vocabulary Assessment

Word Scramble

Unscramble the following terms and correctly write the words.

1. surmises

____

2. vantanoulio

____

3. hearamenor

____

4. tagetsion

____

5. alioch

____

Matching

Match the term in Part 1 with the correct definition in Part 2.

PART 1

1. nulligravida
2. primigravida
3. nullipara
4. multipara
5. parity
6. gravida
7. gravid

PART 2

a. _____ pregnant

b. _____ a woman who has never given birth to a viable fetus

c. _____ a woman who has never been pregnant

d. _____ a woman who has given birth to more than one viable fetus

e. _____ a pregnant woman

f. _____ pregnancies that resulted in a viable birth

Critical Thinking

Answer these questions on a separate sheet of paper.

1. Create a patient education handout on herpes genitalis.
2. Discuss, in a group, factors that may affect a patient's decision to practice contraception as well as the person's choice of methods of contraception. Develop a possible scenario where factors influenced decisions.

Case Studies

1. On May 11, 1999, at 10:00 a.m., Janet Williams has an appointment in your office. Her pregnancy test is positive and the physician has told her that she is pregnant. She asks you to tell her when she can expect her baby to be born. You apply Nagele's rule, based on information that this patient gives you regarding her last menstrual period, which was March 19. How can you educate this patient to the formula that you are using, and what date will you give for an EDD?

   ____

   ____

   ____

   ____

2. You are the senior medical assistant in an OB-GYN office, and as such, you are responsible for training new employees. Today, you will discuss risk factors for fetal abnormalities with a newly hired medical assistant. How will you explain the complex referred to as TORCH?

   ____

   ____

   ____

   ____

CHARTING EXERCISE

Using the situation described in Case Study #1, please give an example of a chart note you might write following patient teaching.

Document on the Patient's Chart:
- Date and time
- Notification of physician
- Patient complaints/concerns
- Patient education
- Your signature

Date/Time	Conditions/Lab Results Patient Communication

Basic Writing Activities

Fill-in-the-Blanks

1. The age at which a girl begins menses is known as ____________________ and is one of the many signs of puberty.
2. Menstruation usually lasts about __________ days.
3. ____________________ is a condition of unknown etiology in which endometrial tissue is found growing outside of the uterine cavity.
4. After AIDS, ____________________ is the most serious STD.

5. The ______________________ is a diagnostic procedure in which the uterus and uterine tubes are radiographed after the injection of a contrast medium.
6. The primary gonads of the female are the ______________________.

Skill Drills

1. List and describe six common obstetric disorders.

____

____

____

2. List and describe three hormonal contraceptive methods and two barrier contraceptives methods.

____

____

____

3. Explain the difference between a contraction stress test (CST) and a nonstress test (NST).

____

____

____

4. Describe the benefits of HRT in menopausal women.

____

____

____

Innovative Activities

Using Nagele's rule formula (the first day of the last menstrual period [LMP] + 7 days – 3 months + 1 year = EDD), calculate the EDD for the following.

1. LMP 2/3/99

____

____

____

2. LMP 5/20/99

____

____

____

3. LMP 8/18/99

____

____

____

4. LMP 10/28/99

____

____

____

COMPETENCY EVALUATION CHECKLIST

Procedure 21-1 Assisting With a Pelvic Examination With a Pap Smear

NAME ______________________ **DATE/TIME** ______________

EVALUATED ______________________ **SCORE** ______________

Goal—To assist with a pelvic examination with a Pap smear.

Objectives/Conditions—When assigned to assist with a pelvic examination with a Pap smear, and equipment and supplies are obtained, the student will appropriately demonstrate how to assist with this type of examination.

Outcome—Assisting with a pelvic examination with a Pap smear will be performed in accordance with the steps presented in the text.

Equipment and Supplies

patient drape
vaginal speculum, appropriate size
uterine sponge forceps
cotton-tipped applicators, long
water-soluble solution
direct lighting
cleansing tissue or personal wipes
biohazard barrier devices, as appropriate
materials for Pap smear—cervical spatula or cervical brush, glass slides, fixative solution (spray or liquid), laboratory request form, identification label
special packaging for safe specimen transport or mailing to the laboratory

Steps	**Y**	**N**	**Number of Attempts**
1. Wash your hands.	☐	☐	______
2. Assemble the equipment and supplies.	☐	☐	______
3. Label and date each slide.	☐	☐	______
4. Complete the laboratory request form for Pap smear with essential information, including the date, patient's name, age, first day of last menstrual period, relevant history, physician, and your signature.	☐	☐	______
5. Greet and identify the patient. Explain the procedure.	☐	☐	______
6. Ask the patient to empty her bladder and if necessary collect a urine specimen.	☐	☐	______
7. Provide the patient with a drape, and ask her to disrobe from the waist down.	☐	☐	______
8. Position the patient in the dorsal lithotomy position with buttocks at the bottom edge of the table.	☐	☐	______
9. Adjust the drape to cover the patient's abdomen and knees, exposing only the genitalia.	☐	☐	______
10. Adjust the light over the genitalia for maximum visibility.	☐	☐	______

Steps (Continued)	Y	N	Number of Attempts
11. Assist the physician with the examination by handing instruments and supplies as needed. Place the spatula firmly in the physician's hand in a functional position.	☐	☐	______
12. Hold the microscopic slides by the frosted ends while the physician is obtaining and making the vaginal and endocervical smears.	☐	☐	______
13. Spray each slide with fixative or immerse each slide in a fixative solution.	☐	☐	______
14. Explain to the patient that the physician will now remove the vaginal speculum and do a bimanual examination of the pelvis.	☐	☐	______
15. Hold a basin for receiving the now contaminated vaginal speculum. Place the speculum in a basin of cold water to begin sanitization.	☐	☐	______
16. Apply about 1 to 2 inches of water-soluble lubricant across the physician's two gloved fingers.	☐	☐	______
17. After completion of the examination, assist the patient in sliding up to the top of the examination table.	☐	☐	______
18. Assist the patient in removing both feet at the same time from the stirrups. Help the patient to remove excess lubricant by handing her a personal wipe or tissues.	☐	☐	______
19. Package the specimen for transport to the laboratory.	☐	☐	______
20. Provide for privacy while the patient is dressing.	☐	☐	______
21. Thank the patient. Reinforce the physician's instructions about follow-up. Address any concerns or questions.	☐	☐	______
22. Properly care for or dispose of equipment. Clean the examination room. Wash your hands.	☐	☐	______

☐ **Pass** ☐ **Fail**

Comments

____

____

____

____

Procedure 21-2 Assisting With Colposcopy With Cervical Biopsy

NAME ______________________ **DATE/TIME** ______________

EVALUATED ______________________ **SCORE** ______________

Goal—To assist with colposcopy with cervical biopsy.

Objectives/Conditions—When assigned to assist with a colposcopy with cervical biopsy, and equipment and supplies are obtained, the student will appropriately demonstrate how to assist with this type of examination.

Outcome—Assisting with a colposcopy with cervical biopsy will be performed in accordance with the steps presented in the text.

Equipment and Supplies

Setup for pelvic examination
Colposcope
Specimen container with preservative (10% formalin)
Sterile gloves
Povidone-iodine (Betadine)
Sanitary napkin, mini pad, or tampon
Biohazard barrier devices, as appropriate
Silver nitrate sticks of ferric subsulfate (Monsel's solution)

On the Sterile Field
Long cotton applicators, sterile
Normal saline solution
3% acetic acid or vinegar
Uterine dressing forceps
Sterile 4×4 gauze
Sterile towel

Sterile Materials for Cervical Biopsy
Biopsy forceps or punch
Uterine curettes
Endocervical curette
Uterine tenaculum

Steps	Y	N	Number of Attempts
1. Verify that the patient has signed the consent form.	☐	☐	______
2. Wash your hands.	☐	☐	______
3. Assemble the equipment and supplies.	☐	☐	______
4. Check the light on the colposcope.	☐	☐	______
5. Set up the sterile field.	☐	☐	______
6. Pour normal saline and acetic acid into their respective sterile containers. Cover the field with a sterile drape.	☐	☐	______
7. Greet and identify the patient. Explain the procedure. Caution the patient that there may be a sharp cramp at the time of biopsy. Have the patient disrobe from the waist down and cover with a privacy drape.	☐	☐	______
8. Position the patient in the dorsal lithotomy position. *Note:* If you are to assist the physician from the sterile field, put on sterile gloves now and assist as follows.	☐	☐	______

Steps (Continued)	**Y**	**N**	**Number of Attempts**
9. Hand the physician the applicator immersed in normal saline, followed by the applicator immersed in acetic acid.	☐	☐	______
10. Hand the physician the applicator with the antiseptic solution (Betadine).	☐	☐	______
11. If you did not glove to assist the physician, put on nonsterile gloves before accepting the specimen.	☐	☐	______
12. Receive the tissue specimen by holding the container of 10% formalin in which the specimen can be immersed.	☐	☐	______
13. Label the specimen container with the patient's name, date, and medical record number.	☐	☐	______
14. Prepare the specimen for transport to the laboratory/pathology.	☐	☐	______
15. Provide the physician with Monsel's solution or silver nitrate sticks, if necessary.	☐	☐	______
16. Explain to the patient that a small amount of bleeding may occur. Have a sanitary pad available.	☐	☐	______
17. Thank the patient. Reinforce the physician's instructions.	☐	☐	______
18. Properly care for or dispose of equipment and supplies. Clean the examination room. Wash your hands.	☐	☐	______

☐ **Pass** ☐ **Fail**

Comments

____

____

____

____

Procedure 21-3 Assisting With the Insertion of an Intrauterine Device

NAME ______________________ **DATE/TIME** ______________

EVALUATED ______________________ **SCORE** ______________

Goal—To assist with the insertion of an intrauterine device.

Objectives/Conditions—When assigned to assist with the insertion of an intrauterine device, and equipment and supplies are obtained, the student will appropriately demonstrate how to assist with this type of examination.

Outcome—Assisting with the insertion of an intrauterine device will be performed in accordance with the steps presented in the text.

Equipment and Supplies

setup for pelvic examination
sterile gloves for the physician and medical assistant
biohazard container
patient drape
sanitary pad
cleansing tissues or personal wipes
biohazard barrier devices, as appropriate
scissors

On the Sterile Field

uterine tenaculum
uterine sound
antiseptic solution (Betadine)
container for solution
sterile transfer forceps
scissors
sterile 4x4 gauze
IUD insertion kit

Steps	Y	N	Number of Attempts
1. Verify that the patient has signed the consent form.	☐	☐	______
2. Wash your hands.	☐	☐	______
3. Prepare equipment and supplies as needed for the pelvic examination (see Procedure 21-1).	☐	☐	______
4. Greet and identify the patient. Explain the procedure. Have the patient disrobe from the waist down and cover with a privacy drape.	☐	☐	______
5. Position and drape the patient in the dorsal lithotomy position, as you would for the pelvic examination.	☐	☐	______
6. Put on gloves or use sterile transfer forceps. Set up the sterile field using strict sterile technique.	☐	☐	______
7. Pour antiseptic solution into the sterile container on the sterile field.	☐	☐	______
8. Assist the physician as directed with gloving and gowning. Adjust the light source over the genitalia.	☐	☐	______

Steps (Continued)	Y	N	Number of Attempts
9. Open the IUD insertion kit with sterile technique. Drop it onto the sterile field, or allow the physician to grasp it from the opened package. The physician will insert the IUD at this point.	☐	☐	______
10. Have scissors available for the physician.	☐	☐	______
11. Assist the patient back up on the table, and help her remove her legs from the stirrups.	☐	☐	______
12. Provide the patient with cleansing tissues or personal wipes.	☐	☐	______
13. Instruct the patient on how and when to check for IUD placement.	☐	☐	______
14. Have the patient check for the placement of the IUD before leaving the office.	☐	☐	______
15. Offer the patient a sanitary pad for small amounts of bleeding that may occur.	☐	☐	______
16. Thank the patient. Reinforce the physician's instructions regarding follow-up and side effects. (If there are no problems, a follow-up visit should be within 4–6 weeks.)	☐	☐	______
17. Properly care for or dispose of equipment and supplies. Clean the room. Wash your hands.	☐	☐	______

☐ Pass ☐ Fail

Comments

____

____

____

____

Procedure 21-4 Assisting With Removal of an Intrauterine Device

NAME ______________________ **DATE/TIME** ______________

EVALUATED ______________________ **SCORE** ______________

Goal—To assist with removal of an intrauterine device.

Objectives/Conditions—When assigned to assist with the removal of an intrauterine device, and equipment and supplies are obtained, the student will demonstrate appropriately how to assist with this type of examination.

Outcome—Assisting with the removal of an intrauterine device will be performed in accordance with the steps presented in the text.

Equipment and Supplies

gloves
patient drape
vaginal speculum
uterine dressing forceps
direct lighting
cleansing tissues or personal wipes
sanitary pad or tampon

Steps	Y	N	Number of Attempts
1. Wash your hands.	☐	☐	______
2. Set up equipment and supplies as for the pelvic examinations (see Procedure 21-1).	☐	☐	______
3. Greet and identify the patient. Explain the procedure. Have the patient disrobe from the waist down and cover with a privacy drape.	☐	☐	______
4. Position the patient in the dorsal lithotomy position.	☐	☐	______
5. Glove and assist the physician as required—adjust the light source, hand the instruments, and receive the contaminated materials on tray or basin.	☐	☐	______
6. Assist the patient back up on the table, and remove her legs from the stirrups.	☐	☐	______
7. Offer the patient a sanitary pad or tampon.	☐	☐	______
8. Thank the patient. Reinforce the physician's instructions.	☐	☐	______
9. Properly care for or dispose of equipment and supplies. Clean the examination room. Wash your hands.	☐	☐	______

☐ Pass ☐ Fail

Comments

____

____

____

____

Procedure 21-5 Assisting With the Insertion of Subdermal Hormonal Implants

NAME ______________________ **DATE/TIME** ______________

EVALUATED ______________________ **SCORE** ______________

Goal—To assist with the insertion of subdermal hormonal implants.

Objectives/Conditions—When assigned to assist with the insertion of subdermal hormonal implants, and equipment and supplies are obtained, the student will demonstrate appropriately how to assist with this type of examination.

Outcome—Assisting with the insertion of subdermal hormonal implants will be performed in accordance with the steps presented in the text.

Equipment and Supplies

sterile gloves for the physician and medical assistant
sterile towel
light source
local anesthetic
patient drape
Norplant system kit (completely self contained with all essential materials)

Additional Materials on the Sterile Field

antiseptic solution
sterile container for antiseptic
sterile syringe (3 or 5 mL)
sterile needle (1 inch, 23–25 gauge)
sterile 4x4 gauze

Steps	Y	N	Number of Attempts
1. Verify that the patient has signed the consent form. Make sure the patient understands all aspects of the procedure.	☐	☐	______
2. Wash your hands.	☐	☐	______
3. Position the patient in the supine position with the chosen upper arm exposed.	☐	☐	______
4. Assemble the equipment and supplies.	☐	☐	______
5. Set up the sterile field.	☐	☐	______
6. Pour antiseptic solution. (*Note:* Antiseptic solution can be poured into the sterile container on the field *or* onto 4 × 4 sterile gauze that remains on top of the inside of the packaging.)	☐	☐	______
7. Open and drop gauze, syringe, and needle onto the field.	☐	☐	______
8. Open the Norplant System and drop onto the field.	☐	☐	______
9. Be aware that the physician may prefer to administer the local anesthetic before gloving. However, if he or she prefers to inject after gloving, follow these steps:			
10. Cleanse the top of the anesthetic vial with alcohol prep.	☐	☐	______

Steps (Continued)	Y	N	Number of Attempts
11. Hold the anesthetic vial in the physician's preferred position while the physician aspirates the anesthetic into the syringe.	☐	☐	________
12. Assist the physician as necessary during the implant insertion.	☐	☐	________
13. Help the patient into an upright position.	☐	☐	________
14. Thank the patient. Reinforce the physician's instructions.	☐	☐	________
15. Properly care for or dispose of equipment and supplies. Clean the room. Wash your hands.	☐	☐	________

☐ **Pass** ☐ **Fail**

Comments

____

____

____

____

22

Pediatric Patients

COMPETENCY PRACTICE

Vocabulary Assessment

Matching

Match the disease in Part 1 with the appropriate immunization in Part 2. Answers from Part 2 may be used more than once.

PART 1	PART 2
1. measles	a. _____ MMR
2. polio	b. _____ OPV
3. mumps	c. _____ DPT
4. diphtheria	d. _____ HBV
5. rubella	e. _____ Hib
6. whooping cough	
7. Hemophilus influenza	
8. tetanus	
9. hepatitis	

Definitions

Write a term for each definition.

1. ________________________ appliance that increases the moisture content in the air
2. ________________________ abnormalities, either structural or functional, that are present from birth
3. ________________________ drawing in or out by suction; as in breathing objects into the respiratory tract or suctioning substances from a site
4. ________________________ viral infection manifested by characteristic rash of successive crops of vesicles that scab before resolution; also called chicken pox
5. ________________________ visit for evaluation of growth and development
6. ________________________ pediatrician that specializes in care of the newborn
7. ________________________ existing or functioning independently
8. ________________________ act or process of rendering an individual immune to a specific disease

Critical Thinking

1. Explain five safety tips you can give parents about giving oral medication to their children.

____

____

____

2. Explain the difference between a well child visit and a sick child visit.

____

____

____

CASE STUDIES

1. John B. is 6 months old and has had a fever for 24 hours and a cough for 3 days. His mother brings him to the pediatrician's office because she has been unable to reduce the fever with Tylenol. John's mother is very concerned because 2 months previously John was hospitalized with pneumonia and she is afraid this will happen again. How can you involve John's mother in the examination to decrease her anxiety?

____

____

____

2. Mary E. is 2 months old and is ready to begin her immunizations. Mary's mother is anxious and wants to know what Mary will be receiving and what to expect after the injections. With regard to the DPT immunization, what can you tell Mary's mother about possible side effects and what she can do for Mary?

____

____

____

CHARTING EXERCISE

With regard to Case Study #2, write a chart note documenting your interaction with Mary's mother.

Document on the Patient's Chart:

- Date and time
- Notification of physician
- Patient complaints/concerns
- Patient education
- Your signature

Date/Time	Conditions/Lab Results Patient Communication

Basic Writing Activities

Skill Drills

1. List five safety precautions that should be followed in a pediatrician's office.

____

____

____

2. List one indicator for each of the following categories of signs of child abuse:
   a. obvious indicators

   ____

   b. hidden indicators

   ____

   c. behavioral indicators

   ____

3. List the common anthropometric measurements obtained in a pediatrician's office.

____

____

____

4. List six factors that can influence a child's temperature.

____

____

____

Short Answer

1. Indicate which temperature method may be used under the following circumstances.
   a. child over 5 to 6 years of age, not seriously ill, septic, and cooperative

   ____

   b. *should not be used* if child is vomiting

   ____

   c. *should not be used* if child has diarrhea

   ____

   d. most readily accepted method by all ages

   ____

2. Children under the age of 2 years old should have their pulses taken

____

____

____

3. Give an example of how each of the following feelings may be expressed by a child during a visit to the pediatrician's office.
   a. fear

   ____

   b. anxiety

   ____

   c. curiosity

   ____

4. Identify a consideration with regard to the development of a child that a medical assistant should make for each of the following age groups.
   a. infancy

   ____

   b. toddler

   ____

   c. preschool

   ____

   d. school-age

   ____

   e. adolescent

   ____

Innovative Activities

Labeling

Plot the following data on an appropriate growth chart.

1. Female child, 36 months old, 30 pounds, 35 inches tall
2. Female child, 10 months old, 16 pounds, 23 inches tall, head circumference 44 cm

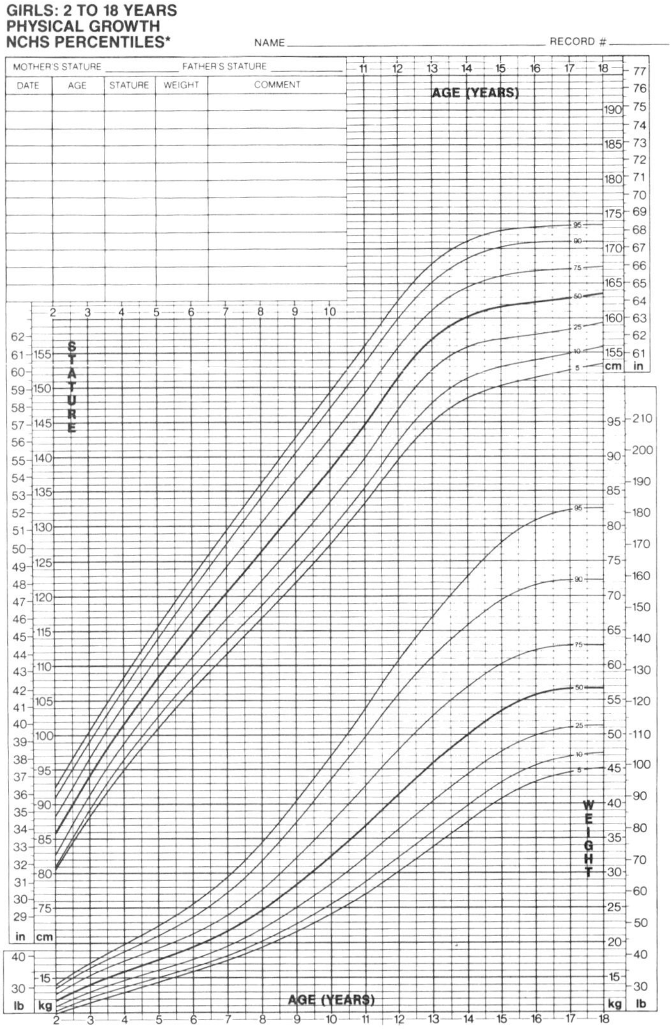

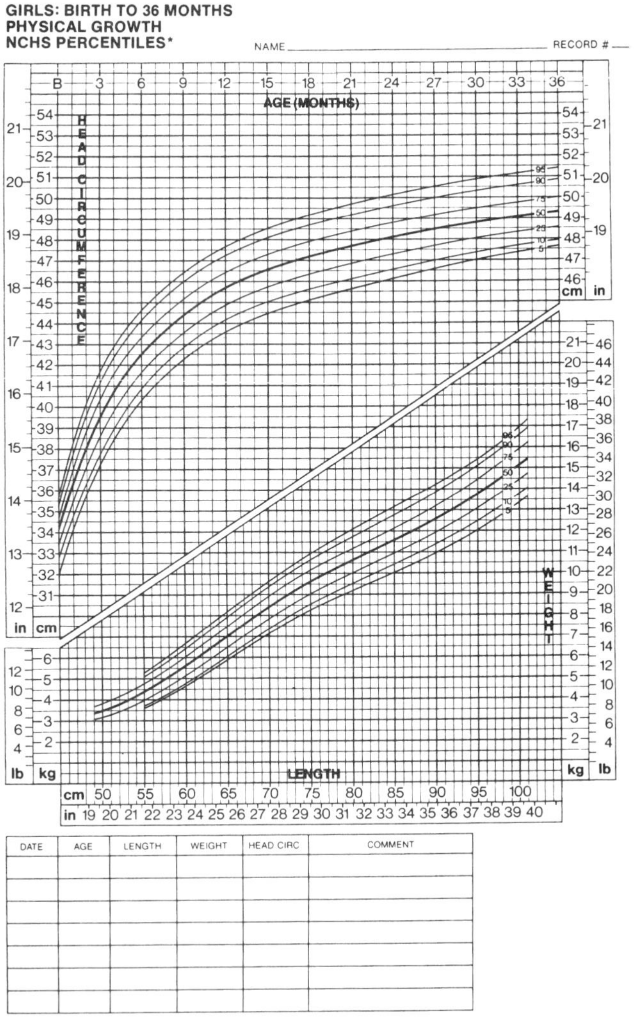

(Adapted from Hamill, P. V. V., Drizd, T. A., Johnson, C. L., Reed, R. B., Roche, A. F., Moore, W. M. [1979]. Physical growth: National Center for Health Statistics percentiles. *Am J Clin Nutr 32;* 607–629. Data from the National Center for Health Statistics [NCHS], Hyattsville, Maryland [Part A]. Data from the Fels Longitudinal Study, Wright State University School of Medicine, Yellow Springs, Ohio [Part B]. Used with permission of Ross Products Division, Abbott Laboratories, Inc. Columbus, OH 43216. © 1993 Ross Products Division, Abbott Laboratories, Inc.)

COMPETENCY EVALUATION CHECKLIST

Procedure 22-1 Restraining a Pediatric Patient

NAME ______________________ **DATE/TIME** ______________

EVALUATED ______________________ **SCORE** ______________

Goal To restrain a pediatric patient.

Objectives/Conditions—When given equipment and supplies listed in the text, the student will safely restrain a pediatric patient.

Outcome—The student will safely restrain a pediatric patient in accordance with the steps in the text.

Equipment and Supplies

Receiving blanket (if using mummy restraint)

Steps	Y	N	Number of Attempts
1. Wash your hands.	☐	☐	______
2. Identify the patient.	☐	☐	______
3. Explain the purpose of the restraint to the child's parents.	☐	☐	______
4. Approach the child in a calm and purposeful manner. Speak softly close to the child's ear.	☐	☐	______
5. Restrain the child using one of these methods.			
a. If only physical restraint is required, stabilize the child's joints.	☐	☐	______
b. If a mummy restraint is required, follow these steps:	☐	☐	______
(1) Place the child diagonally on a small receiving blanket.	☐	☐	______
(2) Wrap the left corner across the torso, covering the right arm and shoulder. Pull it snugly under the child's left arm and tuck it under the child's body.	☐	☐	______
(3) Pull the right corner across the child's left arm and shoulder and tuck it snugly under the torso at the back so that the child's weight secures the end.	☐	☐	______
(4) Tuck the bottom of the blanket around the child.	☐	☐	______
6. Guard against excessive pressure on the area of the child's body that is being restrained.	☐	☐	______
7. Observe the child for any signs of respiratory distress or pain. Adjust the restraint or the holding position as necessary.	☐	☐	______
8. Wash your hands.	☐	☐	______

☐ Pass ☐ Fail

Comments

____

____

____

____

Procedure 22-2 Measuring Height

NAME ______________________ DATE/TIME ______________

EVALUATED ______________________ SCORE ______________

Goal—To measure height.

Objectives/Conditions—When given equipment and supplies listed in the text, the student will measure height.

Outcome—The student will accurately measure height in accordance with the steps in the text.

Equipment and Supplies

Wall-mounted measuring unit
Growth chart

Steps	Y	N	Number of Attempts
1. Wash your hands.	☐	☐	______
2. Greet and identify the child.	☐	☐	______
3. Explain the procedure to the parent or to the child in an age-appropriate manner.	☐	☐	______
4. Measure the child's height.	☐	☐	______
5. Praise the child for cooperating.	☐	☐	______
6. Record the child's height on the growth chart and in the patient chart.	☐	☐	______
7. Wash your hands.	☐	☐	______

☐ Pass ☐ Fail

Comments

____

____

____

____

Procedure 22-3 Measuring Length

NAME ______________________ **DATE/TIME** ______________

EVALUATED ______________________ **SCORE** ______________

Goal—To measure length.
Objectives/Conditions—When given equipment and supplies listed in the text, the student will measure length.
Outcome—The student will accurately measure length in accordance with the steps in the text.

Equipment and Supplies

Examining table with clean paper
Tape measure or measuring board
Growth chart
Pencil

Steps	Y	N	Number of Attempts
1. Wash your hands.	☐	☐	______
2. Identify the patient.	☐	☐	______
3. Place the child on a firm examining table covered with clean paper. If using a measuring board, cover with clean paper.	☐	☐	______
4. Measure the child's length:			
a. Fully extend the child's body by holding the head in the midline.	☐	☐	______
b. Grasp the knees and gently press flat onto the table.	☐	☐	______
c. Mark the top of the head and the heel of the feet on the paper.	☐	☐	______
d. Have the parent pick up the child or move the child away from the section of the paper used for measuring.	☐	☐	______
e. Measure between the marks in either inches or centimeters, or read the measurement indicated on the measuring board if this is the method used.	☐	☐	______
5. Record the child's length on the growth chart and in the patient chart.	☐	☐	______
6. Wash your hands.	☐	☐	______

☐ Pass ☐ Fail

Comments

____
____
____
____

Procedure 22-4 Measuring Chest and Head Circumference

NAME ______________________ ______________________ **DATE/TIME** ______________________

EVALUATED ______________________ **SCORE** ______________________

Goal—To measure chest and head circumference.
Objectives/Conditions—When given equipment and supplies listed in the text, the student will measure chest and head circumference.
Outcome—The student will accurately measure chest and head circumference in accordance with the steps in the text.

Equipment and Supplies

Paper or cloth measuring tape
Growth chart

Steps	Y	N	Number of Attempts
1. Wash your hands.	☐	☐	______
2. Identify the patient.	☐	☐	______
3. Place the child supine on the examining table, or ask the parent to hold the child.	☐	☐	______
4. Measure around the chest at the nipple line, keeping the measuring tape at the same level anteriorly and posteriorly.	☐	☐	______
5. Measure around the head above the eyebrow and posteriorly at the largest part of the occiput.	☐	☐	______
6. Record the child's chest and head circumference on the growth chart and in the patient chart.	☐	☐	______
7. Wash your hands.	☐	☐	______
Note: If chest and head growth are within normal limits, these measurements usually are not required after 12 months.	☐	☐	______

☐ Pass ☐ Fail

Comments

____

____

____

____

Procedure 22-5 Measuring Weight

NAME ______________________ **DATE/TIME** ______________

EVALUATED ______________________ **SCORE** ______________

Goal—To measure weight.
Objectives/Conditions—When given equipment and supplies listed in the text, the student will measure weight.
Outcome—The student will accurately measure weight in accordance with steps in the text.

Equipment and Supplies

Infant scale
Protective paper for the scale
Growth chart

Steps	Y	N	Number of Attempts
1. Wash your hands.	☐	☐	______
2. Identify the child.	☐	☐	______
3. Explain the procedure to the parent or to the child in an age-appropriate manner.	☐	☐	______
4. Place a protective paper on the scale.	☐	☐	______
5. Balance the scale.	☐	☐	______
6. Follow these steps to weigh an infant:			
a. Place the infant gently on the scale, or have the parent place the infant.	☐	☐	______
b. Know that infants are weighed lying down.	☐	☐	______
c. Keep in mind that children who can sit may be weighed in a sitting position if this is less frightening for them.	☐	☐	______
d. Have the parent stand in the child's view.	☐	☐	______
e. Keep one of your hands near the child at all times.	☐	☐	______
f. Just before balancing the scale, remove an infant's diaper. *Note:* Wear gloves to handle diapers, as feces have been implicated in the transmission of disease. (Children may leave on undergarments while being weighed.)	☐	☐	______
g. Balance the scale quickly but carefully, moving the counterbalances to the proper places on the weight bar to balance the apparatus exactly.	☐	☐	______
h. Have the parent pick up and soothe the child.	☐	☐	______

Steps (Continued)	Y	N	Number of Attempts
7. Record the child's weight on the growth chart and in the patient chart.	☐	☐	______
8. Wash your hands.	☐	☐	______

☐ **Pass** ☐ **Fail**

Comments

____

____

____

____

Procedure 22-6 Measuring Pediatric Blood Pressure

NAME ____________________ **DATE/TIME** ____________

EVALUATED ____________________ **SCORE** ____________

Goal—To measure a pediatric blood pressure.

Objectives/Conditions—When given equipment and supplies listed in the text, the student will measure a pediatric blood pressure.

Outcome—The student will accurately measure a pediatric blood pressure in accordance with steps in the text.

Equipment and Supplies

Stethoscope
Sphygmomanometer

Steps	Y	N	Number of Attempts
1. Wash your hands.	☐	☐	______
2. Select the appropriate size cuff.	☐	☐	______
3. Identify the patient.	☐	☐	______
4. Explain the procedure to the child's parent or to the child in an age-appropriate manner. For instance, you might say, "This may squeeze your arm a little bit."	☐	☐	______
5. Expose the child's arm and determine the systolic pulse as described for adults. (See Chap. 3, Anthropometric Measurements and Vital Signs.)	☐	☐	______
6. Wrap the cuff around the arm 1/2 to 1 inch above the antecubitus.	☐	☐	______
7. Place the chest piece of the stethoscope at the antecubital area. Pump the cuff about 30 mm Hg above the last pulse felt.	☐	☐	______
8. Release the pressure 2–4 mm Hg per second and note the first return of the pulse. This will be the systolic measurement. Note the last sound heard; this will be the diastolic pressure.	☐	☐	______
9. Thank the child for cooperating.	☐	☐	______
10. Care for the equipment as appropriate.	☐	☐	______
11. Wash your hands.	☐	☐	______

☐ **Pass** ☐ **Fail**

Comments

____

____

____

____

Procedure 22-7 Applying a Pediatric Urine Collection Device

NAME ______________________________ **DATE/TIME** ______________

EVALUATED ______________________________ **SCORE** ______________

Goal—To apply a pediatric urine collection device.
Objectives/Conditions—When given equipment and supplies listed in the text, the student will apply a pediatric urine collection device.
Outcome—The student will apply a pediatric urine collection device in accordance with steps in the text.

Equipment and Supplies

Personal antiseptic wipes or cotton balls and antiseptic solution
Pediatric urine collection bag
Completed laboratory request slip
Transport container

Steps	Y	N	Number of Attempts
1. Wash your hands.	☐	☐	______
2. Assemble the equipment and supplies.	☐	☐	______
3. Identify the patient.	☐	☐	______
4. Explain the procedure to the child's parents.	☐	☐	______
5. Place the child in a supine position and ask for help from the parent, as needed.	☐	☐	______
6. Put on gloves.	☐	☐	______
7. Clean the genitalia with the wipes or solution.	☐	☐	______
a. For females: Cleanse front to back with separate wipes for each downward stroke on the outer labia. The last clean wipe should be between the inner labia (or labia minora).	☐	☐	______
b. For males: Retract the foreskin if the baby has not been circumcised, if possible. Cleanse the meatus in an ever-widening circle. Discard the wipe and repeat. Return the foreskin to position.	☐	☐	______
8. Holding the collection device, remove the upper portion of the paper backing and press it around the mons pubis. Remove the second section and press it against the perineum. Loosely attach the diaper.	☐	☐	______
9. Give the baby fluids unless contraindicated, and check the diaper frequently for the specimen.	☐	☐	______
10. When the child has voided, remove the device, clean the skin of residual adhesive, and rediaper.	☐	☐	______
11. Perform a routine urinalysis (see Chap. 28, Urinalysis), or route the specimen as required.	☐	☐	______
12. Remove gloves and wash your hands.	☐	☐	______

☐ **Pass** ☐ **Fail**

Comments

____

____

____

____

23

Geriatric Patients

COMPETENCY PRACTICE

Vocabulary Assessment

Matching

Match the definition in Part 1 with the correct term in Part 2.

PART 1

1. acute episodes of cerebrovascular insufficiency
2. mental deterioration
3. abnormally slow voluntary movements
4. farsightedness
5. whirling sensation
6. lens opacity
7. hearing loss

PART 2

a. _____ bradykinesia

b. _____ vertigo

c. _____ presbycusis

d. _____ transient ischemic attacks

e. _____ dementia

f. _____ presbyopia

g. _____ cataracts

Definitions

Define the following terms.

1. syncope

____

____

____

2. lentigines

____

____

____

3. activities of daily living (ADLs)

____

____

____

4. keratoses (senile)

____

____

____

5. biotransforming

____

____

____

6. dysphagia

____

____

____

7. positron emission tomography (PET)

____

____

____

Critical Thinking

1. Compare and contrast active neglect and passive neglect as they relate to elder abuse.

____

____

____

2. Describe the responsibility of the medical assistant in relation to elder abuse.

____

____

____

Case Studies

1. Mrs. Ellison is 85 years old. She has been a widow for 10 years. During that time she has lived alone without incident. Mrs. Ellison recently sustained a series of falls. Although she has not been seriously injured, her family, that lives 200 miles away, is concerned for her safety. With regard to other living arrangements, what are the options for Mrs. Ellison?

____

____

____

2. Mr. Jones, aged 62, has been diagnosed with Alzheimer's disease. Mr. Jones's daughter has accompanied him to the office for a routine examination. While Mr. Jones is being examined, his daughter expresses her concern and frustration with the progression of the disease. She states that she is exhausted most of the time yet feels she cannot leave her father alone. What can you say to Mr. Jones's daughter? What advice may you offer?

____

____

____

CHARTING EXERCISE

With regard to Case Study #2, write a narrative chart note describing your interaction with the patient and his family.

Document on the Patient's Chart:

- Date and time
- Notification of physician
- Patient complaints/concerns
- Patient education
- Your signature

Date/Time	Conditions/Lab Results Patient Communication

Basic Writing Activities

Skill Drills

1. List four approaches you might use to reinforce medical compliance in the elderly.

____

____

____

2. List five common risk factors for elder abuse.

____

____

____

3. Describe the seven signs of suicidal intent.

____

____

____

4. List three medications that may be prescribed for patients with Parkinson's disease.

____

____

____

Fill-in-the-Blanks

1. _______________ is a slow, progressive disease thought to be caused by a loss of dopamine in the brain cells.
2. Threatening an elder with imprisonment or physical abuse, withholding food or medication, or physical isolation are examples of _______________ abuse.
3. Symptoms of Alzheimer's disease may appear as early as age _______________.
4. Maintaining optimum health in the elderly should focus on the areas of _______________ and _______________.
5. Elderly patients should be counseled to *increase* their intake of _______________, _______________, and _______________.
6. Elderly patients should be counseled to *decrease* their intake of _______________, _______________, and _______________.
7. _______________ and _______________ are two age-related barriers to understanding explanations about medications.

24

Diagnostic Imaging

COMPETENCY PRACTICE

Vocabulary Assessment

Matching

Match the definition in Part 1 with the correct term in Part 2.

PART 1

1. x-rays and computers create cross-sectional image of the body
2. high frequency sound waves create cross-sectional image of the body
3. observe movement within the body
4. magnetic field, radio waves, and computers create cross-sectional image of the body
5. "cameras" and radionuclides create an image
6. specialized x-ray of the breast

PART 2

a. _____ MRI

b. _____ CT scan

c. _____ mammography

d. _____ nuclear medicine

e. _____ sonography

f. _____ fluoroscopy

Definitions

Define the following terms.

1. cassette

____

____

2. radiograph

____

____

3. radiography

____

____

4. radiologist

____

____

5. radiopaque

____

____

Critical Thinking

Answer these questions on a separate sheet of paper.

1. Give legal tips to a new employee regarding x-ray procedures, in order to safeguard the patient and employees.

____

____

____

2. What can you tell a patient about how to prevent constipation following a barium enema?

____

____

____

Case Studies

1. Dr. Reed has ordered a chest x-ray for Mrs. Adams as part of her annual physical examination. Dr. Reed has an x-ray unit in the office and on the way to the x-ray room Mrs. Adams asks you about the dangers of x-rays. How will you respond?

____

____

____

2. Mr. Hersch is a 53-year-old man who is scheduled for an upper GI series. Mr. Hersch is concerned about the discomfort he believes will occur during the examination. He has had abdominal pain for 2 months and is worried that the test will reveal an ulcer. He wonders if he will have to take medication or have surgery. Mr. Hersch has many questions and appears visibly anxious. What steps can the medical assistant take to alleviate Mr. Hersch's anxiety?

____

____

____

CHARTING EXERCISE

Using the situation described in Case Study #2, write a narrative chart note describing your interaction with the patient.

Document on the Patient's Chart:

- Date and time
- Notification of physician
- Patient complaints/concerns
- Patient education
- Your signature

Date/Time	Conditions/Lab Results Patient Communication

Basic Writing Activities

Skill Drills

1. List the seven responsibilities of the medical assistant during the performance of a routine radiographic examination.

____

____

____

2. List five radiation safety procedures directed toward patients.

____

____

____

3. Identify three ways the medical assistant directly assists the patient during the radiographic examination.

____

____

____

Fill-in-the-Blanks

1. The _______________________ records the amount of radiation to which a worker has been exposed.
2. Percutaneous transluminal coronary angioplasty is also known as _______________________.
3. _______________________ use laser beams to remove deposits in vessels.
4. Unexposed film must be protected from moisture, heat, and _______________________.

Innovative Activities

Labeling

Identify and label the different x-ray positions.

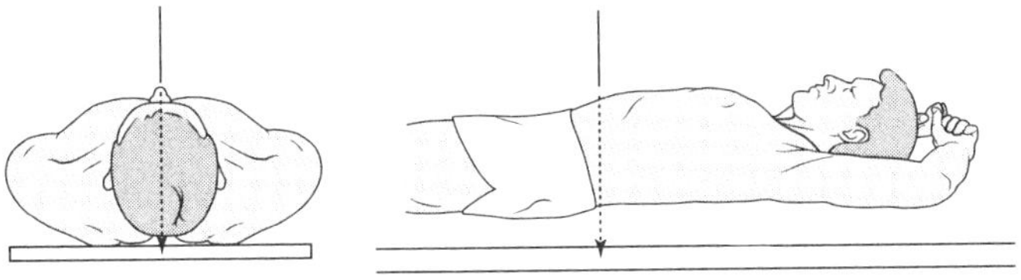

____

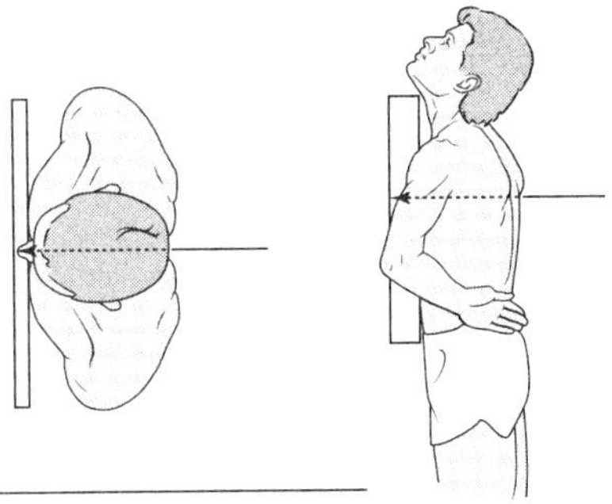

____

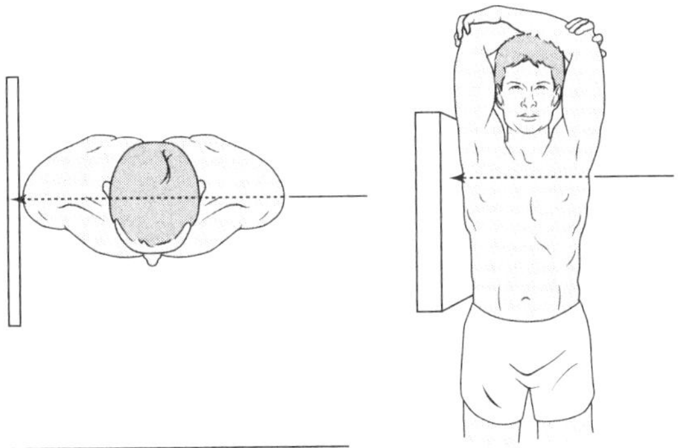

____

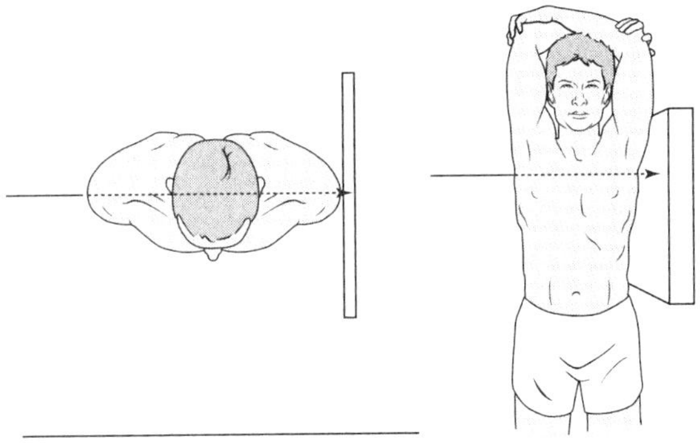

____

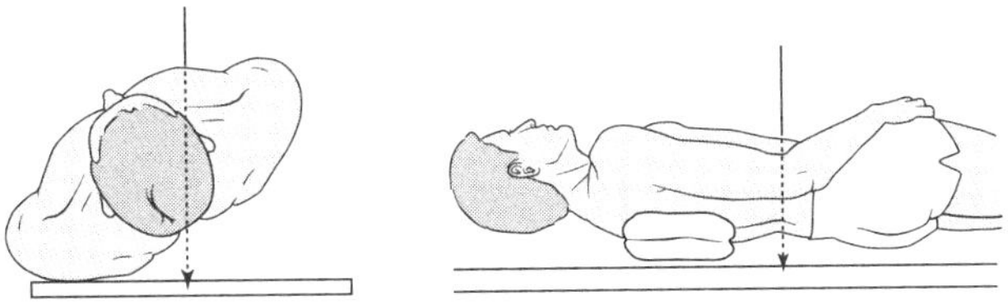

____

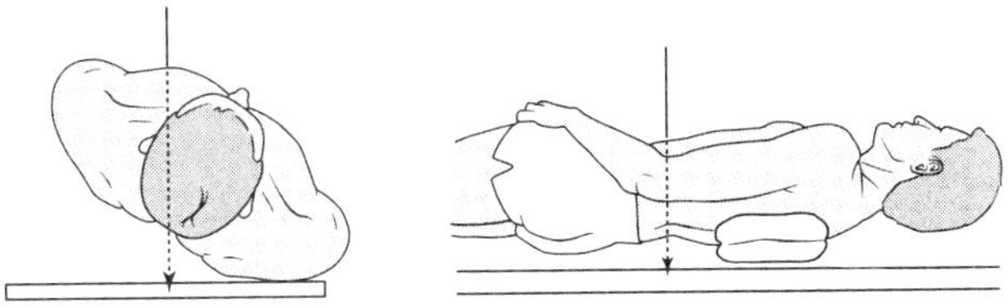

____

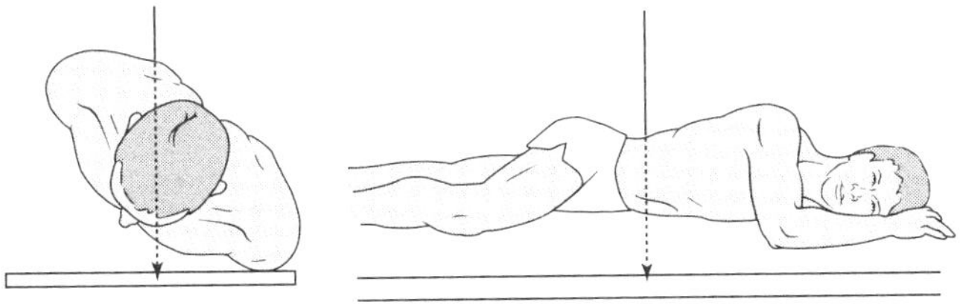

____

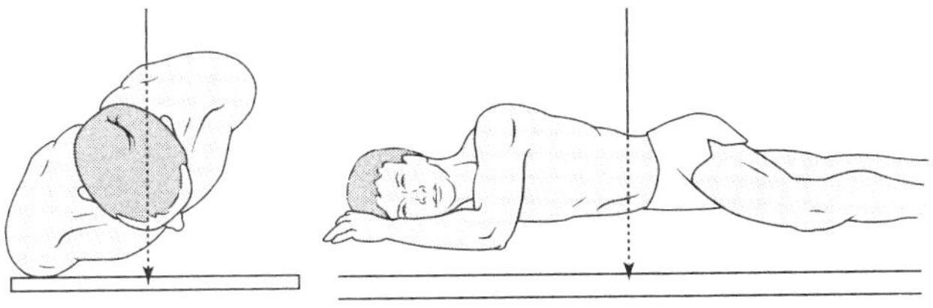

____

25

Medical Office Emergency

COMPETENCY PRACTICE

Vocabulary Assessment

Fill-in-the-Blanks

Fill-in the blanks with the term defined in each sentence.

1. a severe system reaction resulting from an allergic reaction

   ____

2. an accumulation of blood at a bruise site that causes the skin to become black and blue

   ____

3. a blood clot at an injury site

   ____

4. the involuntary contraction of voluntary muscles; an abnormal discharge of electrical activity in the brain

   ____

5. a type of shock that is caused by a generalized infection in the body

   ____

6. body temperature below normal

   ____

Matching

Match the definition in Part 1 with the correct term in Part 2.

PART 1

1. third-degree burn
2. loss of blood or other body fluid
3. first-degree burn
4. dysfunction of the nervous system
5. second-degree burn
6. rapid evaluation to determine patient's status
7. left ventricle cannot pump blood to body

PART 2

a. _____ superficial burn

b. _____ neurogenic shock

c. _____ cardiogenic shock

d. _____ full-thickness burn

e. _____ primary survey

f. _____ hypovolemic shock

g. _____ partial-thickness burn

Critical Thinking

1. Allan is a 16-year-old boy who fell off his bicycle 30 minutes ago. According to his mother, he may have been unconscious for an undetermined amount of time. She has brought Allan to Dr. Lee's office for an examination. You know that the pupils can provide important clues to the neurological status of patients. All trauma patients and those who have sustained head injuries should have their pupils checked. Explain how Dr. Lee will examine the pupils and the five items that should be evaluated.

____

____

____

2. It is lunch time at the medical office where you work. Your co-worker has already started eating when you enter the break room. Suddenly, your co-worker cannot speak and clutches at her throat. What do you think may be happening? How would you assess the situation and what would your first action be?

____

____

____

Case Studies

1. Allison is an 18-year-old patient of Dr. Armstrong. She has just seen Dr. Armstrong for a physical examination before she leaves for college in the northeast. Allison's hobby is mountain climbing and she enthusiastically tells you about plans for a mountain climb in November. As the office Medical Assistant, what can you tell Allison about the effects of hypothermia and how to protect herself from frostbite?

____

____

____

2. You are the supervising medical assistant in an emergency clinic. The Medical Director asks you to deliver an inservice to the other staff on types of shock. What will you tell the staff about the various types and management of shock?

____

____

____

CHARTING EXERCISE

Using the situation described in Case Study #1, give an example of a chart note you might write following patient teaching.

Document on the Patient's Chart:

- Date and time
- Notification of physician
- Patient complaints/concerns
- Patient education
- Your signature

Date/Time	Conditions/Lab Results Patient Communication

Basic Writing Activities

Fill-in-the-Blanks

1. The ________________ is the most common method of determining the extent of burn injuries.
2. A ________________ is the medical term for heart attack.
3. An ________________ is a substance that gives rise to hypersensitivity or allergy.
4. ________________ refers to the general condition of excess body heat.
5. The primary goal of therapy in the patient with a severe anaphylactic reaction is to restore ________________ and ________________ function.
6. An ________________ is the tearing loose of a flap of skin, which may either remain hanging or tear off altogether.

Skill Drills

1. List three types of hyperthermic emergencies and the treatment of each one.

____

____

____

2. List the seven components of an emergency action plan.

____

____

____

3. List the eight management guidelines for burn victims.

____

____

____

4. Describe the universal sign for distress in choking.

____

____

____

Innovative Activities

Labeling

Identify and label the percentage assigned to each body part shown on the adult and child figures according to the rule of nines.

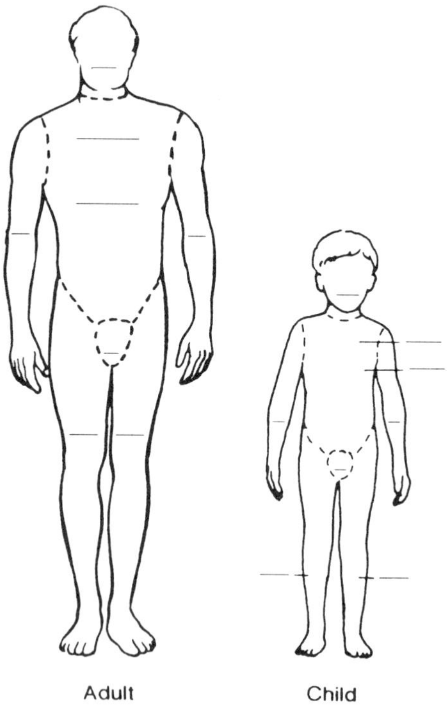

COMPETENCY EVALUATION CHECKLIST

Procedure 25-1 Managing an Adult Patient With a Foreign Body Airway Obstruction (FBAO)

NAME ______________________________ **DATE/TIME** ______________

EVALUATED ______________________________ **SCORE** __________

Goal—To restore airway patency by removing a foreign body obstruction.

Objectives/Conditions—When presented with a simulated FBAO scenario, the student will demonstrate (in simulation) the appropriate management of an adult with a foreign body airway obstruction and identify needed equipment and supplies.

Outcome—Management of an FBAO will be performed in accordance with the steps presented in the text.

Equipment and Supplies

barrier respiratory devices
gloves

Steps	Y	N	Number of Attempts
1. Ask the patient, "Are you choking?" If the patient is able to speak or cough, the obstruction is not complete. Observe the patient for increased distress and assist the patient as needed, but do not perform thrusts.	☐	☐	______
2. If the patient is unable to speak or cough and is displaying the universal sign for distress (grasping the throat), follow these steps to perform abdominal thrusts:			
a. Stand behind the patient and wrap your arms around his or her waist.	☐	☐	______
b. Make a first with your nondominant hand, thumb side against the patient's abdomen at midline between navel and xiphoid.	☐	☐	______
c. Grasp the fist with your dominant hand and give quick upward abdominal thrusts. Completely relax your arms between each thrust and make each thrust forceful enough to relieve the obstruction.	☐	☐	______
3. Repeat thrusts until effective or the victim becomes unconscious.	☐	☐	______
4. If the victim is unconscious, or becomes unconscious, activate the EMS system.	☐	☐	______
5. Glove now. Perform a tongue-jaw lift followed by a finger sweep to remove the object.	☐	☐	______
6. Open the airway and try to ventilate. If the airway is still obstructed, reposition the patient's head and try to ventilate again. Use a barrier respiratory device if available.	☐	☐	______

Steps (Continued)	**Y**	**N**	**Number of Attempts**
7. Begin abdominal thrusts:			
a. Straddle the patient's hips.	☐	☐	______
b. Place the long axis of your nondominant palm between the patient's navel and xiphoid process.	☐	☐	______
c. Lace your fingers with the dominant hand against the back of the properly positioned non-dominant hand.	☐	☐	______
d. Give up to five upward abdominal thrusts.	☐	☐	______
8. Repeat steps 5 through 7 until effective.	☐	☐	______

☐ **Pass** ☐ **Fail**

Comments

____

____

____

____

Procedure 25-2 Performing Cardiopulmonary Resuscitation (One Rescuer)

NAME ______________ ______________ **DATE/TIME** ______________

EVALUATED ______________ **SCORE** ______________

Goal—To maintain or restore cardiopulmonary function after cardiac arrest until emergency services are available.

Objectives/Conditions—When presented with a simulated adult cardiac arrest scenario, the student will correctly demonstrate one-rescuer CPR (in simulation) and identify needed equipment and supplies.

Outcome—CPR (in simulation) will be performed in accordance with the steps presented in the text.

Equipment and Supplies

barrier respiratory devices
gloves

Steps	Y	N	Number of Attempts
1. Establish patient unresponsiveness by shaking the patient and shouting "Are you okay?"	☐	☐	______
2. Activate the EMS system if there is no response.	☐	☐	______
3. Place the patient in the supine position with head level with the body. Kneel by his shoulders.	☐	☐	______
4. Open the airway with the head-tilt/chin-lift maneuver.	☐	☐	______
5. Determine breathlessness by looking, listening, and feeling for breaths.	☐	☐	______
6. If the patient is breathing and his or her condition allows, place the patient in the recovery position (refer to Fig. 25-7) until consciousness returns or help arrives.	☐	☐	______
7. If the patient is not breathing, maintain head-tilt/chin-lift and give two slow breaths just until the chest rises.	☐	☐	______
8. Check the carotid pulse.	☐	☐	______
9. If no pulse is present, follow these steps to perform chest compression:			
a. Locate the costal–xiphoid (xiphocostal) notch.	☐	☐	______
b. Place the long axis of the nondominant palm on the sternum two fingers above the costal–xiphoid notch.	☐	☐	______
c. Lace the fingers with the dominant hand pressing against the back of the nondominant hand at the proper position.	☐	☐	______
d. With your upper body perpendicular to the patient's chest, rock from the hips with the force of the upper body and stiffened arms, compressing the sternum 1 1/2 to 2 inches.	☐	☐	______
e. Keep your hands in position during the upstroke, but allow the patient's chest to expand completely before the next compression. Give cycles of 15 chest compressions and two breaths at a rate of 80 to 100 per minute.	☐	☐	______

Steps (Continued)	Y	N	Number of Attempts
10. After giving four cycles of 15 chest compressions and 2 breaths (about 1 minute), check the patient's carotid pulse. If no pulse is present, continue the 15:2 cycle beginning with chest compressions. Continue until help arrives or until a pulse is present at the pulse check. If the pulse returns but respirations do not, continue giving breaths at 14 to 16 per minute until help arrives. Transport the patient to an emergency facility.	☐	☐	______

☐ **Pass** ☐ **Fail**

Comments

____

____

____

____

26

Introduction to the Clinical Laboratory

COMPETENCY PRACTICE

Vocabulary Assessment

Matching

Match the definition in Part 1 with the correct term in Part 2.

PART 1

1. sorts specimens and enters data
2. performs on large, automated instruments
3. collects and processes blood samples
4. helps manage test result information
5. answers phones and tracks specimens
6. large facility performing tests
7. primarily inpatient tests

PART 2

a. _____ technologist

b. _____ customer service personnel

c. _____ hospital laboratory

d. _____ reference laboratories

e. _____ accessioners

f. _____ phlebotomist

g. _____ secretaries

Definitions

Define the following terms.

1. calibration

____

____

____

2. capillary action

____

____

____

3. centrifugal force

____

____

____

4. material safety data sheet (MSDS)

5. normal value

6. reagent

7. specimen

Critical Thinking

1. You are asked to educate other staff in laboratory safety and today you will discuss ways to avoid spills. What will you tell the staff?

2. You have been asked to draw a CBC. What type of personal protective equipment will you use, and why?

CASE STUDIES

1. Dr. Walters has ordered a CBC and a UA for Mr. Marks. Lab request forms need to be filled out and sent to Universal Labs. You know that certain types of information will be necessary to complete the forms. Please explain.

2. Dr. Williams has ordered a blood glucose test for Ms. Cochran. The patient is anxious about having this test done and asks questions about how the test will be performed, the type of specimen required, and why the test is being performed. As a medical assistant, you know that patient education is important. How will you educate this patient?

CHARTING EXERCISE

Using the situation described in Case Study #1, write a narrative chart note describing your interaction with the patient.

Document on the Patient's Chart:

- Date and time
- Notification of physician
- Patient complaints/concerns
- Patient education
- Your signature

Date/Time	Conditions/Lab Results Patient Communication

Basic Writing Activities

Skill Drills

1. List eight of the most common tests performed in a physician's office laboratory.

____

____

____

2. List seven of the most common reasons for laboratory testing.

____

____

____

3. Name six basic pieces of equipment common to most small laboratories.

____

____

____

4. Name three basic types of hazards in the laboratory and give an example of each.

____

____

____

Fill-in-the-Blanks

1. An ______________________ is anything that prevents or delays blood clotting.
2. ______________________ testing involves measuring blood levels of both therapeutic drugs and drugs of abuse.
3. The study of bacteria is called ______________________.
4. The study of the microscopic structures of tissue is called ______________________.
5. ______________________ involves the study of the microscopic structure of cells.

Innovative Activities

Obtain copies of three material safety data sheets regarding common cleansers and share the information in class.

COMPETENCY EVALUATION CHECKLIST

Procedure 26-1 Caring for a Microscope

NAME ______________________ **DATE/TIME** ______________

EVALUATED ______________________ **SCORE** ______________

Goal—To care for a microscope.
Objectives/Conditions—When asked to demonstrate the correct method of caring for a microscope, the student will obtain appropriate equipment and supplies then demonstrate the required action.
Outcome—A microscope is cleaned in accordance with the steps presented in the text.

Equipment and Supplies

Lens paper
Lens cleaner
Gauze
Mild soap solution
Microscope

Steps	Y	N	Number of Attempts
1. Wash your hands.	☐	☐	______
2. Assemble the equipment.	☐	☐	______
3. If you need to move the microscope, carry it using two hands—one to hold the base and the other to hold the arm.	☐	☐	______
4. Clean the ocular areas, following these steps:			
a. Place a drop or two of lens cleaner on a piece of lens paper. Never use tissue or gauze because these may scratch the ocular areas.	☐	☐	______
b. Wipe each eyepiece thoroughly with the lens paper. To prevent the transfer of oils from your skin, avoid touching the ocular areas with your fingers.	☐	☐	______
c. Wipe each objective lens, starting with the lowest power first and continuing to the highest power (usually an oil immersion lens). If the lens paper appears to have dirt or oil on it, use a clean section of the lens paper, or use a new piece of lens paper with cleaner.	☐	☐	______
d. Using a new piece of lens paper, wipe each eyepiece and objective lens so that no cleaner remains.	☐	☐	______
5. Clean the nonocular areas, following these steps:			
a. Moisten gauze with mild soap and wipe down all nonocular areas, including the stage, base, and adjustment knobs.	☐	☐	______
b. Moisten another gauze with water and rinse the washed areas.	☐	☐	______

Steps (Continued)	Y	N	Number of Attempts
6. To store the cleaned microscope, ensure that the light source is turned off. Rotate the nosepiece so that the low-power objective is pointed down toward the stage. Cover the microscope if appropriate.	☐	☐	__________

☐ **Pass** ☐ **Fail**

Comments

27

Microbiology

COMPETENCY PRACTICE

Vocabulary Assessment

Matching

Match the definition in Part 1 with the correct term in Part 2.

PART 1

1. food poisoning
2. anthrax
3. tetanus
4. gas gangrene
5. athlete's foot
6. ringworm of the body
7. nail fungus

PART 2

a. _____ *Clostridium tetani*

b. _____ tinea pedis

c. _____ *Clostridium botulinum*

d. _____ tinea corporis

e. _____ *Clostridium perfringens*

f. _____ tinea unguium

g. _____ *Bacillus anthracis*

Definitions

Write a term for the following definitions.

1. ________________________ very absorbent
2. ________________________ surgical puncture made into a cavity
3. ________________________ to require; a parasite that has no choice but to attach to a living organism
4. ________________________ stick topped with cotton or other absorbent man-made fiber for cleaning areas, applying treatments, or obtaining specimens
5. ________________________ the study of viruses
6. ________________________ a substance used to fix, or bind, dyes or stains
7. ________________________ a type of seaweed or algae that helps solidify culture media; the media may be referred to as agar

Critical Thinking

1. Describe how culture media plates are to be stored. Why? What should the medical assistant check for before using the plates?

2. What causes streptococcal pharyngitis infections? What are the symptoms? How is it treated?

Case Studies

1. Mary Smith is being seen by Dr. Allan because she has had a fever to 102 (orally) for 2 days and a headache and sore throat for 1 day. Dr. Allan orders a rapid strep test. You collect the specimen and perform the test. It is positive. Mary receives a prescription for amoxicillin 250 mg to be taken four times a day for 10 days. What is a rapid strep test? Why was it ordered?

2. George Smith is being seen for chronic diarrhea. Dr. Adams has the results of a stool culture. It reveals that Mr. Smith is suffering from dysentery. What type of organism would cause dysentery? What type of laboratory would perform the culture?

CHARTING EXERCISE

With regard to Case Study #1, write a narrative chart note describing your actions.

Document on the Patient's Chart:

- Date and time
- Notification of physician
- Patient complaints/concerns
- Patient education
- Your signature

Date/Time	Conditions/Lab Results Patient Communication

Basic Writing Activities

Skill Drills

1. List the four steps in the preparation of a wet mount slide.

2. List the five steps in the preparation of a hanging drop slide.

3. Explain how a Gram stain is a diagnostic tool.

____

____

____

4. State factors that are necessary for microbial growth.

____

____

____

Short Answer

1. Identify the following organisms as fungi (F) or protozoa (P).
   a. Trichomonas ____________________
   b. tinea ____________________
   c. Coccidioides ____________________
   d. Histoplasma ____________________
   e. Giardia ____________________
   f. Aspergillus ____________________
2. For the most reliable results, laboratory tests should be performed within ____________ hour(s) after collection.
3. ____________________ is a process that helps physicians narrow the field of possible pathogens and indicate treatment before a culture has been incubated.
4. Meningitis and botulism are diseases caused by gram-____________________ bacteria.
5. Anaerobic bacteria live without ____________________.
6. Blood agar is a solid medium that is prepared by adding 5% ____________________ blood to agar.
7. A liquid medium for cultures is made of ____________________ and is provided in a small jar or tube.

Innovative Activities

Label Design

Design a label to be attached to every specimen collection that includes all pertinent data.

COMPETENCY EVALUATION CHECKLIST

Procedure 27-1 Properly Labeling and Identifying a Specimen for Transportation and Handling

NAME ______________________ **DATE/TIME** ______________

EVALUATED ______________________ **SCORE** ______________

Goal—To properly label and identify a specimen for transportation and handling.

Objectives/Conditions—When given equipment and supplies listed in the text, the student will properly label and identify a specimen for transportation and handling.

Outcome—The student will properly label and identify a specimen for transportation and handling in accordance with steps in the text.

Equipment and Supplies

Appropriate laboratory requisition
Specimen container/mailing container

Steps	Y	N	Number of Attempts
1. Assemble the equipment.	☐	☐	______
2. Complete the laboratory request form.	☐	☐	______
3. Wash hands and put on gloves.	☐	☐	______
4. Check the expiration date and the condition of the transport medium.	☐	☐	______
5. Peel the envelope away from the transport tube about one-third of the way and remove the tube.	☐	☐	______
6. Label the tube with the date, the patient's name, the source of the specimen, and initials of the person processing the specimen.	☐	☐	______
7. Obtain the specimen as directed by the physician or receive the specimen as the collection procedure is performed by the physician.	☐	☐	______
8. Return the swab to the tube and follow the manufacturer's recommendation for immersion into the medium.	☐	☐	______
9. Remove and dispose of gloves and wash hands.	☐	☐	______
10. Package for transport as directed by the manufacturer's recommendations on the packaging. Some specify returning the tube to the peel-apart envelope.	☐	☐	______
11. Route the specimen.	☐	☐	______

☐ Pass ☐ Fail

Comments

____

____

____

____

Procedure 27-2 Preparing a Dry Specimen Smear

NAME ______________________ **DATE/TIME** ______________

EVALUATED ______________________ **SCORE** ______________

Goal—To prepare a dry specimen smear.
Objectives/Conditions—When given equipment and supplies listed in the text, the student will prepare a dry specimen smear.
Outcome—The student will prepare a dry specimen smear in accordance with steps in the text.

Equipment and Supplies

Specimen
Slide forceps
Sterile swab or inoculating loop
Bunsen burner
Slide
Pencil or diamond-tipped pen

Steps	Y	N	Number of Attempts
1. Wash your hands.	☐	☐	______
2. Assemble the equipment.	☐	☐	______
3. Label the slide with the patient's name and the date on the frosted edge.			
4. Put on gloves and face shield. Hold the edges of the slide between the thumb and index finger. Starting at the right side of the slide and using a rolling motion of the swab or a sweeping motion of the inoculating loop, gently and evenly spread the material from the specimen over the slide. The material should thinly fill the center of the slide within 1/2 inch of each end.	☐	☐	______
5. Do not rub the material vigorously over the slide.	☐	☐	______
6. Dispose of the contaminated swab or inoculating loop in a biohazard container. If you are not using a disposable loop, sterilize it as follows:			
a. Hold the loop in the colorless part of the flame of the Bunsen burner for 10 seconds.	☐	☐	______
b. Raise the loop slowly (to avoid splattering the bacteria) to the blue part of the flame until the loop and its connecting wire glow red.	☐	☐	______
c. If reusing the loop, cool the loop so the heat will not kill the bacteria that must be allowed to grow. Do not wave the loop in the air because doing so may expose it to contamination. Do not stab the medium with a hot loop to cool; this creates an aerosol.	☐	☐	______
7. Allow the smear to air dry in a flat position for at least 1/2 hour. Do not wave it about in the air. Heat should not be applied until the specimen has been allowed to dry. Some specimens require a fixative spray (eg, Pap smears).	☐	☐	______

Steps (Continued)	Y	N	Number of Attempts
8. Hold the dried smear slide with the slide forceps. Pass the slide quickly through the flame of a Bunsen burner three or four times. The slide has been fixed properly when the back of the slide feels slightly uncomfortably warm to the back of the gloved hand. It should not feel hot.	☐	☐	______
9. Examine the smear under the microscope, or stain it according to office policy. In most instances, the physician examines the slide for identification.	☐	☐	______
10. Dispose of equipment and supplies in appropriate containers. Remove and dispose of gloves and wash your hands.	☐	☐	______

☐ **Pass** ☐ **Fail**

Comments

____

____

____

____

Procedure 27-3 Preparing a Specimen With Gram Stain

NAME ______________________ **DATE/TIME** ______________

EVALUATED ______________________ **SCORE** ________

Goal—To prepare a specimen with Gram stain.

Objectives/Conditions—When given equipment and supplies listed in the text, the student will prepare a specimen with Gram stain.

Outcome—The student will prepare a specimen with Gram stain in accordance with steps in the text.

Equipment and Supplies

Crystal violet stain
Gram's iodine solution
Alcohol-acetone solution
Counterstain (eg, Safranin)
Specimen on a glass labeled using a slide diamond-tipped pen
Bunsen burner
Slide forceps
Staining rack
Wash bottle with distilled water
Absorbent (bibulous) paper pad
Immersion oil
Microscope
Stop watch or timer

Steps	Y	N	Number of Attempts
1. Wash your hands.	☐	☐	________
2. Assemble the equipment.	☐	☐	________
3. Make sure that the specimen is heat fixed to the labeled slide and that the slide is room temperature before beginning. (See Procedure 27-2: Preparing a Dry Smear.)	☐	☐	________
4. Put on gloves.	☐	☐	________
5. Place the slide on the staining rack with the smear side upward.	☐	☐	________
6. Flood the smear with crystal violet. Time with the stop watch or timer for 30 to 60 seconds.	☐	☐	________
7. Hold the slide with slide forceps.	☐	☐	________
a. Tilt the slide to an angle of about 45 degrees to drain the excess dye.	☐	☐	________
b. Rinse the slide with distilled water from the wash bottle for about 5 seconds and drain off the excess water.	☐	☐	________
8. Replace the slide on the slide rack. Flood the slide with Gram iodine solution and time for 30 to 60 seconds.	☐	☐	________
9. Using the forceps, tilt the slide at a 45-degree angle to drain iodine solution. With the slide tilted, rinse the slide with distilled water from the wash bottle for about 5 to 10 seconds. Slowly and gently wash with the alcohol–acetone solution until no more purple stain runs off.	☐	☐	________

Steps (Continued)	**Y**	**N**	**Number of Attempts**
10. Immediately rinse the slide with distilled water for 5 seconds and return the slide to the rack.	☐	☐	______
11. Flood with the Safranin or suitable counterstain. Time process for 30 to 60 seconds.	☐	☐	______
12. Drain the excess counterstain from the slide by tilting it at a 45-degree angle.	☐	☐	______
13. Inspect the slide using oil immersion objective lens for greatest magnification. The physician interprets the slide.	☐	☐	______
14. Properly care for or dispose of equipment and supplies. Clean the work area. Remove gloves and wash your hands.	☐	☐	______

☐ **Pass** ☐ **Fail**

Comments

____

____

____

____

Procedure 27-4 Inoculating a Culture and Conduct Sensitivity Testing

NAME ______________________ **DATE/TIME** ______________

EVALUATED ______________________ **SCORE** ______________

Goal—To inoculate a culture and conduct sensitivity testing.

Objectives/Conditions—When given equipment and supplies listed in the text, the student will inoculate a culture and conduct sensitivity testing.

Outcome—The student will inoculate a culture and conduct sensitivity testing in accordance with steps in the text.

Equipment and Supplies

Specimen on a swab or loops
Bunsen burner
China marker or permanent markers
Labeled Petri dish (The patient's name should be on the side of the plate containing the medium, because it is always placed upward to prevent condensation from dripping onto the culture.)

Steps	Y	N	Number of Attempts
1. Assemble the equipment.	☐	☐	______
2. Put on gloves and the face shield.	☐	☐	______
3. Label the plate with the patient's name, identification number, source of specimen, time collected, time inoculated, your initials, and date.	☐	☐	______
4. Remove the Petri plate from the cover (the Petri plate is always stored inverted with the cover downward), and place the cover with the opening upward on the work surface. Do not open the cover unnecessarily.	☐	☐	______
5. Using a rolling and sliding motion, streak the specimen swab completely across 1/2 of the plate starting from the top and working to a midpoint or at the diameter of the plate. Dispose of the swab in a biohazard container. If the inoculating loop is used for lifting a secondary culture, streak in the same manner.	☐	☐	______
6. Dispose of this loop. If your office does not use disposable inoculating loops, sterilize the loop as described in step 6 of Procedure 27-2.	☐	☐	______
7. Turn the plate 1/4 turn from its previous position. Pass the loop a few times in the original inoculum then downward into the media approximately 1/4 of the surface of the plate. Do not enter the originally streaked area after the first few sweeps.	☐	☐	______
8. Dispose of this loop. If you are not using a disposable loop, flame loop and allow it to cool again.	☐	☐	______
9. Turn the plate another 1/4 turn so that now it is 180 degrees to the original smear. Working in the previous manner, draw the loop at right angles through the most recently streaked area. Again, do not enter the originally streaked area after the first few sweeps.	☐	☐	______

Steps (Continued)	**Y**	**N**	**Number of Attempts**
10. If the plate is to be used for sensitivity, follow these steps:			
a. Using sterile forceps or an automatic dispenser, place the specified disks on areas of the plate equidistant from each other.	☐	☐	______
b. Press them gently with the sterilized loop or forceps until good contact is made with the surface of the agar.	☐	☐	______
11. Properly care for or dispose of equipment and supplies. Remove gloves and wash your hands.	☐	☐	______
12. Incubate for the specified period of time. Read the results and record as directed by office policy.	☐	☐	______

☐ **Pass** ☐ **Fail**

Comments

____

____

____

____

28

Urinalysis

COMPETENCY PRACTICE

Vocabulary Assessment

Matching

Match the definition in Part 1 with the correct term in Part 2.

PART 1

1. substance formed from creatine metabolism
2. material composed of particles
3. settling out
4. nitrogenous compounds derived from protein use excreted in urine
5. double nitrogen compound that reacts with bilirubin
6. unit of measurement for urobilinogen
7. enzyme contained in leukocytes

PART 2

a. _____ esterase

b. _____ diazo

c. _____ precipitation

d. _____ creatinine

e. _____ particulate matter

f. _____ urates

g. _____ Ehrlich units

Word Scramble

Unscramble each of the following medical terms.

1. mianoma

____

2. urelcut

____

3. culactifloon

____

4. elsy

____

5. trelolectye

____

Critical Thinking

1. Explain why a 24-hour urine collection is used to detect such proteins as creatine and electrolytes.

____

____

____

2. Patients are often asked to give a clean-catch midstream urine specimen. How will you explain this type of urine collection to patients?

____

____

____

Case Studies

1. Mr. Wheatherby is a 70-year-old man with a history of congestive heart failure who has a routine appointment with Dr. Davies this afternoon. Prior to Mr. Wheatherby's appointment, the physician instructs you to obtain a urine specimen from the patient when he arrives, and to run a specific gravity on the urine. When this patient arrives you give him a urine specimen container and ask him to try to urinate a little into the cup. Once you have obtained the specimen you take it into the lab area and test for specific gravity using a refractometer. You find the specific gravity to be 1.030. Considering Mr. Wheatherby's medical history, why do you think Dr. Davies asked for a urine specific gravity. What is the normal specific gravity range?

____

____

____

2. Mrs. Smith has experienced three episodes of urinary tract infection in the past 2 months. Today she is seeing Dr. Alexander for what she believes to be a recurrence of the UTI she had 3 weeks previously. Mrs. Smith tells you that she would like to use the restroom before she sees the doctor. Considering Mrs. Smith's history and her symptoms today, would you have her collect a urine specimen? If a specimen is to be collected, what type would it be? Explain.

____

____

____

CHARTING EXERCISE

Using the situation described in Case Study #1, write a narrative chart note describing your interaction with the patient, including the collection of a urine specimen.

Document on the Patient's Chart:

- Date and time
- Notification of physician
- Patient complaints/concerns
- Patient education
- Your signature

Date/Time	Conditions/Lab Results Patient Communication

Basic Writing Activities

Skill Drills

1. List three types of examinations of urine that comprise a complete urinalysis.

____

____

____

2. List four conditions that can cause bleeding in the urinary tract, evidenced by hematuria.

____

____

____

3. List six conditions that can cause proteins to appear in urine.

____

____

____

4. List six disorders that can be detected by an examination of urine.

____

____

____

Fill-in-the-Blanks

Complete the following sentences.

1. Once urine is collected, testing should be done within ______________.
2. The presence and multiplication of microorganisms in an unrefrigerated urine specimen changes the pH from acidic to ______________.
3. Other than a CCMS, an aseptic urine specimen can be collected through ______________.
4. Glucose is filtered and reabsorbed in the ______________.
5. Ketones are a group of chemicals that result from ______________.

Innovative Activities

Write examples of possible causes next to the given color and clarity of urine from Table 28-1.

Table 28–1 **Common Causes for Variations in the Color and Clarity of Urine**

Color/Clarity	*Possible Causes*
Yellow-brown or green-brown	
Dark yellow or orange	
Bright orange-red	
Red or reddish-brown	
Brownish-black	
Black	
Grayish or smokey	
Cloudy	

Note: In addition to the causes noted above, foods such as blackberries, rhubarb, beets, and those with red dye are common causes of dark or reddish urine that might resemble hematuria.

COMPETENCY EVALUATION CHECKLIST

Procedure 28-1 Obtaining a Clean Catch Midstream (CCMS) Urine Specimen

NAME ______________________ **DATE/TIME** ____________

EVALUATED ______________________ **SCORE** ____________

Goal—To obtain a CCMS urine specimen.

Objectives/Conditions—When asked to obtain a clean catch midstream urine specimen, the student will gather appropriate supplies and correctly instruct the patient in the collection technique.

Outcome—A CCMS is obtained, using correct patient instructions, supplies, equipment, and handling techniques in accordance with the steps presented in the text.

Equipment and Supplies

Sterile cotton balls or appropriate antiseptic wipes
Antiseptic (if using cotton balls)
Sterile water
Sterile urine container labeled with patient's name
Bedpan or urinal (if necessary)

Steps	Y	N	Number of Attempts
1. Wash your hands. If you are to assist the patient, put on gloves.	☐	☐	______
2. Assemble the equipment.	☐	☐	______
3. Identify the patient and explain the procedure. Ask for and answer any questions.	☐	☐	______
4. If the patient is to perform the procedure, provide the necessary supplies.	☐	☐	______
5. Have the patient perform the procedure.	☐	☐	______
a. *Instruct the male patient to:*			
(1) Expose the glans penis by retracting the foreskin, then clean the meatus with a cotton ball or wipe soaked in a mild antiseptic or a towelette. The glans should be cleaned in a circular motion away from the meatus. A new wipe should be used for each cleaning sweep.	☐	☐	______
(2) Keeping the foreskin retracted, void the first 30 mL into the toilet or urinal.	☐	☐	______
(3) Bring the sterile container into the urine stream and collect a sufficient amount (about 30–100 mL). Instruct the patient to avoid touching the inside of the container with the penis.	☐	☐	______
(4) Finish voiding into the toilet or urinal.	☐	☐	______

Steps (Continued)	Y	N	Number of Attempts
b. *Instruct the female patient to:*			
(1) Kneel or squat over a bedpan or toilet bowl. Spread the labia minor widely to expose the meatus. Using cotton balls soaked in a mild antiseptic or wipe, cleanse on either side of the meatus then the meatus itself. Use a wipe or cotton ball only once in a sweep from the anterior to the posterior surfaces, then discard it. Rinse with cotton balls soaked in sterile water in the same manner.	☐	☐	______
(2) Keeping the labia separated, void the first 30 mL into the toilet.	☐	☐	______
(3) Bring the sterile container into the urine stream and collect a sufficient amount (about 30–100 mL).	☐	☐	______
(4) Finish voiding into the toilet or bedpan.	☐	☐	______
6. Recap the filled container and drop it into the outside carry container or place it in a designated area.	☐	☐	______
7. Properly care for or dispose of equipment and supplies. Clean the work area. Remove gloves and wash your hands.	☐	☐	______

☐ **Pass** ☐ **Fail**

Comments

____

____

____

____

Procedure 28-2 Explaining the Method of Obtaining a 24-Hour Urine Specimen

NAME ______________________ **DATE/TIME** ______________

EVALUATED ______________________ **SCORE** ______________

Goal—To explain the method of obtaining a 24-hour urine specimen.

Objectives/Conditions—When asked to explain the method of obtaining a 24-hour urine specimen, the student will gather appropriate supplies and equipment and correctly explain the method of obtaining a 24-hour urine specimen.

Outcome—An explanation of the method of obtaining a 24-hour urine specimen is given, in accordance with the steps presented in the text.

Equipment and Supplies

Patient's labeled 24-hour urine container (some patients may require more than one container)
Preservatives required for the specific test
Hazard labels
Volumetric cylinder (holds at least 1 L)
Serologic or volumetric pipettes
Clean random urine container
Fresh 10% bleach solution
Patient log form

Steps	Y	N	Number of Attempts
1. Wash your hands.	☐	☐	________
2. Assemble the equipment.	☐	☐	________
3. Identify the type of 24-hour urine collection requested and check for any special requirements, such as any acid or preservative that should be added. Label the container appropriately.	☐	☐	________
4. Put on gloves and PPE.	☐	☐	________
5. Add the correct amount of acid or preservative, if needed, using a serologic or volumetric pipette to the 24-hour urine container.	☐	☐	________
6. Use a label provided or write on the 24-hour urine container "Beginning Time ____ and Date ____" and "Ending Time ____ and Date ____" so that the patient can fill in the appropriate information.	☐	☐	________
7. Instruct the patient to collect a 24-hour urine sample as follows:	☐	☐	________
a. Void into the toilet, and note this time and date as "beginning."	☐	☐	________
b. After the first voiding, collect each voiding and add it to the urine container for the next 24 hours.	☐	☐	________
c. Precisely 24 hours after beginning collection, empty the bladder even if there is no urge to void.	☐	☐	________
d. Note on the label the "ending" time and date.	☐	☐	________

Steps (Continued)	Y	N	Number of Attempts
8. Explain to the patient that, depending on the test requested, the 24-hour urine may need to be refrigerated the entire time. Instruct the patient to return the specimen to you as soon as possible after collection is complete.	☐	☐	______
9. Record in the patient's chart that supplies and instructions were given to collect a 24-hour urine specimen and the test that was requested.	☐	☐	______
10. After receiving the 24-hour urine specimen from the patient, verify beginning and ending times and dates before the patient leaves. Check for required acids or preservatives that need to be added before routing the specimen to the laboratory, if applicable.	☐	☐	______
11. Pour the urine into a cylinder to record the total volume collected during the 24-hour period. Pour a small representative sample (aliquot) of the urine into a clean container to be sent to the laboratory. (Label the specimen with a biohazard label if this is not prominently displayed on the container.) Record the volume of the urine collection and the amount of acid or preservative added (if needed) on the sample container and on the laboratory requisition. If permissible, you may dispose of the remainder of the urine.	☐	☐	______
12. Record the volume on the patient log form.	☐	☐	______
13. Clean the cylinder with fresh 10% bleach solution, then rinse with water. Let it air dry.	☐	☐	______
14. Clean the work area and dispose of waste properly. Remove PPE and wash your hands.	☐	☐	______

☐ **Pass** ☐ **Fail**

Comments

____

____

____

____

Procedure 28-3 Determining Urine Color and Clarity

NAME ______________________ **DATE/TIME** ______________

EVALUATED ______________________ **SCORE** __________

Goal—To determine urine color and clarity.

Objectives/Conditions—When asked to determine urine color and clarity, the student will obtain appropriate supplies and equipment and correctly determine urine color and clarity.

Outcome—The color and clarity of urine is determined in accordance with the steps presented in the text.

Equipment and Supplies

Patient's labeled urine specimen
Clear glass tube, usually a centrifuge
White paper scored with black lines

Steps	Y	N	Number of Attempts
1. Wash your hands.	☐	☐	______
2. Assemble the equipment.	☐	☐	______
3. Put on gloves, gown, and face shield.	☐	☐	______
4. Verify that the names on the specimen container and the laboratory form are the same.	☐	☐	______
5. Pour 10–15 mL of urine into the tube.	☐	☐	______
6. In bright light, examine the urine for color. The most common colors are straw (very pale yellow), yellow, dark yellow, and amber (brown-yellow). Other colors include blue, green, red, orange, brown, and black.	☐	☐	______
7. Determine urine clarity. Hold the urine tube in front of the white paper scored with black lines. If the lines are seen clearly (not obscured), record as clear. If the lines are seen but are not well delineated, record as hazy. If the lines cannot be seen at all, record as cloudy.	☐	☐	______
8. Properly care for or dispose of equipment and supplies. Clean the work area. Remove gloves, gown, and face shield. Wash your hands.	☐	☐	______

☐ Pass ☐ Fail

Comments

____

____

____

____

Procedure 28-4 Determining Specific Gravity of Urine by Urinometer

NAME ______________________ **DATE/TIME** ______________

EVALUATED ______________________ **SCORE** ______________

Goal—To test the specific gravity of urine using a urinometer.

Objectives/Conditions—When asked to test the specific gravity of urine using a urinometer, the student will obtain appropriate equipment and supplies and correctly demonstrate this procedure.

Outcome—The specific gravity of urine is tested correctly using a urinometer in accordance with the steps presented in the text.

Equipment and Supplies

Patient's labeled urine specimen
Urinometer with cylinder (Note: Urinometers also are known as hydrometers.)
Patient report form
Kemwipe or clean paper towel

Steps

Steps	Y	N	Number of Attempts
1. Wash your hands.	☐	☐	______
2. Assemble the equipment.	☐	☐	______
3. Put on impervious gown, gloves, and face shield.	☐	☐	______
4. Verify that the names on the specimen container and the laboratory form are the same.	☐	☐	______
5. Make sure the urinometer is clean before beginning. Use distilled water and a Kemwipe or paper towel to wipe the inside of the cylinder and urinometer free of lint and moisture.	☐	☐	______
6. Add the patient's well-mixed, room-temperature urine specimen to the cylinder until it is two thirds full.	☐	☐	______
7. Add the urinometer to the cylinder with a spinning motion.	☐	☐	______
8. Read the specific gravity of the urine specimen from the urinometer scale. Observe the value from the bottom of the meniscus.	☐	☐	______
9. Record the value on the patient's report form and in the patient's chart.	☐	☐	______
10. With a Kemwipe or paper towel, wipe the urinometer dry after the testing procedure.	☐	☐	______
11. Clean the work area, and dispose of waste properly. Remove gown, gloves, and face shield. Wash your hands.	☐	☐	______

☐ Pass ☐ Fail

Comments

____

____

____

____

Procedure 28-5 Determining Specific Gravity of Urine by Refractometer

NAME ______________________ **DATE/TIME** ______________

EVALUATED ______________________ **SCORE** ______________

Goal—To test the specific gravity of urine using a refractometer.

Objectives/Conditions—When asked to test the specific gravity of urine using a refractometer, the student will obtain appropriate equipment and supplies and correctly demonstrate this procedure.

Outcome—The specific gravity of urine is tested correctly using a refractometer in accordance with the steps presented in the text.

Equipment and Supplies

Patient's labeled urine specimen
Transfer pipettes
Refractometer
Kemwipe or clean gauze
Light source

Steps	Y	N	Number of Attempts
1. Wash your hands.	☐	☐	______
2. Assemble the equipment.	☐	☐	______
3. Verify that the names on the specimen container and the laboratory form are the same.	☐	☐	______
4. Put on impervious gown, gloves, and face shield.	☐	☐	______
5. Make sure the refractometer is clean before beginning. Use distilled water and a Kemwipe or gauze to wipe the cover and the prism clean and free of moisture.	☐	☐	______
6. Using a clean pipette, place a drop of the patient's well-mixed, room-temperature urine onto the notch of the cover. (If the urine has been refrigerated, allow it to reach room temperature because cold affects specific gravity readings.) The urine should flow over the prism.	☐	☐	______
7. Point the refractometer toward a light source, and observe the level where the dark and the light portions meet. Record the patient's specific gravity on the worksheet and in the patient's chart.	☐	☐	______
8. Wipe the refractometer clean with distilled water and dry with a gauze or Kemwipe. *This prepares the instrument for the next use.*	☐	☐	______
9. Clean the work area and dispose of waste properly. Remove PPE and wash your hands.	☐	☐	______

☐ Pass ☐ Fail

Comments

____

____

____

____

Procedure 28-6 Accurately Interpreting Chemical Reagent Strip Reactions

NAME ______________________ **DATE/TIME** ______________

EVALUATED ______________________ **SCORE** ____________

Goal—To accurately interpret a chemical reagent strip reaction.

Objectives/Conditions—When asked to interpret a chemical reagent strip reaction, the student will obtain appropriate supplies and equipment and correctly demonstrate how to interpret the reaction.

Outcome—A chemical reagent strip reaction is accurately interpreted in accordance with the steps presented in the text.

Equipment and Supplies

Patient's labeled urine specimen
Chemical strip (such as Multistix or Chemstrip)
Manufacturer's color comparison chart
Stopwatch or timer

Steps	Y	N	Number of Attempts
1. Wash your hands.	☐	☐	______
2. Assemble the equipment.	☐	☐	______
3. Put on gloves, impervious gown, and face shield.	☐	☐	______
4. Verify that the names on the specimen container and the laboratory form are the same.	☐	☐	______
5. Mix the patient's urine by gently swirling the covered container.	☐	☐	______
6. Remove the reagent strip from its container, and replace the lid to prevent deterioration of strips by humidity.	☐	☐	______
7. Immerse the reagent strip in the urine completely, then immediately remove it, sliding the side edge of the strip along the lip of the urine container to remove excess urine from the pads.	☐	☐	______
8. Start your stopwatch or timer immediately.	☐	☐	______
9. Compare the reagent pad areas to the color chart, determining results at the intervals stated by the manufacturer. Example: Glucose is read at 30 seconds. To determine results, examine that pad at 30 seconds post-dipping, and compare with color chart for glucose.	☐	☐	______
10. Read all reactions at the times indicated and record results.	☐	☐	______

Steps (Continued)	Y	N	Number of Attempts
11. Discard the reagent strips in the proper receptacle. Discard urine unless more testing is required.	☐	☐	________
12. Clean the work area. Remove gown, gloves, and face shield. Wash your hands.	☐	☐	________

☐ **Pass** ☐ **Fail**

Comments

Procedure 28-7 Performing a Copper Reduction Test for Glucose

NAME ______________________ **DATE/TIME** ______________

EVALUATED ______________ ______________ **SCORE** __________

Goal—To perform a copper reduction test for glucose.

Objectives/Conditions—When asked to perform a copper reduction test for glucose, the student will obtain appropriate supplies and equipment and correctly demonstrate how this test is performed.

Outcome—A copper reduction test for glucose is performed in accordance with the steps presented in the text.

Equipment and Supplies

Patient's labeled urine specimen
Positive and negative controls
Clinitest tablets (tightly sealed or new bottle)
16 × 125 mm glass test tubes
Test tube rack
Transfer pipettes
Distilled water
Stopwatch or timer
Five-drop Clinitest color comparison chart
Daily sample log
Patient report form and data form

Steps	Y	N	Number of Attempts
1. Wash your hands.	☐	☐	______
2. Assemble the equipment.	☐	☐	______
3. Put on impervious gown, gloves, and face shield.	☐	☐	______
4. Identify the patient's specimen to be tested, and record patient and sample information on the daily log.	☐	☐	______
5. Record the patient's name or identification information, catalog and lot numbers for all test and control materials, and expiration dates on report or data form.	☐	☐	______
6. Label test tubes with patient sample identification or as controls, and place them in the test tube rack.	☐	☐	______
7. Using a transfer pipette, add 10 drops of distilled water to each labeled test tube in the rack. Add drops by holding the dropper vertically to ensure proper delivery.	☐	☐	______
8. Add 5 drops of the patient's urine or control sample to the appropriately labeled tube, using a different transfer pipette for each.	☐	☐	______
9. Open the Clinitest bottle, and shake a Clinitest tablet into the lid without touching it. Then drop the tablet from the lid into the sample in the test tube rack. Repeat for all patient and control samples being tested. Close the Clinitest bottle.	☐	☐	______
10. Observe reactions in the test tubes as the mixture boils. After the reaction stops, wait 15 seconds, then gently shake the test tubes.	☐	☐	______

Steps (Continued)	Y	N	Number of Attempts
11. Compare the results for the patient specimen and controls with the 5-drop method color chart immediately after shaking. (If positive or negative controls do not give expected results, the test is invalid and must be repeated.)	☐	☐	______
12. Clean and disinfect the work area, and dispose of all waste properly. Remove gown, gloves, and face shield. Wash your hands.	☐	☐	______

☐ **Pass** ☐ **Fail**

Comments

____

____

____

____

Procedure 28-8 Performing Nitroprusside Reaction (Acetest) for Ketones

NAME ______________________ **DATE/TIME** ______________

EVALUATED ______________________ **SCORE** ______________

Goal—To perform a nitroprusside reaction test (Acetest) for ketones.

Objectives/Conditions—When asked to perform a nitroprusside reaction (Acetest) for ketones, the student will obtain appropriate supplies and equipment and correctly demonstrate how this test is performed.

Outcome—A nitroprusside reaction (Acetest) for ketones is performed in accordance with the steps presented in the text.

Equipment and Supplies

Patient's labeled urine specimen
White filter paper
Plastic transfer pipette
Acetest tablet
Manufacturer's color comparison chart

Steps	Y	N	Number of Attempts
1. Wash your hands.	☐	☐	________
2. Assemble the equipment.	☐	☐	________
3. Put on gloves, impervious gown, and face shield.	☐	☐	________
4. Place an Acetest tablet on the filter paper by shaking one into the cap and dispensing it onto the paper. Replace the cap.	☐	☐	________
5. Using a transfer pipette, place 1 drop of well-mixed urine on top of the tablet.	☐	☐	________
6. Wait 30 seconds for the complete reaction.	☐	☐	________
7. Compare the color of the tablet to the color chart, and record the results as negative, trace, small amount, moderate amount, or large amount.	☐	☐	________
8. Properly care for or dispose of equipment and supplies. Clean the work area. Remove gloves, gown, and face shield, and wash hands.	☐	☐	________

☐ Pass ☐ Fail

Comments

____

____

____

____

Procedure 28-9 Performing an Acid Precipitation Test

NAME ______________________ **DATE/TIME** ______________

EVALUATED ______________________ ______________ **SCORE** __________

Goal—To perform an acid precipitation test.

Objectives/Conditions—When asked to perform an acid precipitation test, the student will obtain appropriate equipment and supplies, and correctly demonstrate how this test is performed.

Outcome—An acid precipitation test is performed in accordance with the steps presented in the text.

Equipment and Supplies

Patient's labeled and centrifuged urine specimen
Positive and negative controls
3% sulfosalicylic acid (SSA) solution
Clear glass test tubes
Test tube rack
Transfer pipettes
Stopwatch or timer
Daily sample log
Patient report form or data form

Steps	Y	N	Number of Attempts
1. Wash your hands.	☐	☐	______
2. Assemble the equipment.	☐	☐	______
3. Put on impervious gown, gloves, and face shield.	☐	☐	______
4. Identify the patient's specimen to be tested, and record patient and sample information on the daily log.	☐	☐	______
5. Record the patient's name or identification information, catalog and lot numbers for all test and control materials, and expiration dates on report or data form.	☐	☐	______
6. Label the test tubes with patient sample identification or as controls, and place in test tube rack.	☐	☐	______
7. Centrifuge at 1,500 RPM for 5 minutes.	☐	☐	______
8. Add 1 to 3 mL of supernatant urine (top portion of spun urine) or control sample to appropriately labeled tube in rack. Repeat for all samples and controls, using a clean transfer pipette for each. (*Note:* If supernatant from centrifuged urine is not used or the specimen is not mixed after centrifugation, a false-positive result may occur.)	☐	☐	______
9. Add an equal amount of 3% SSA solution to sample quantity in each tube. Use a clean transfer pipette for each addition if your 3% SSA solution does not have a repeating dispenser.	☐	☐	______
10. Mix the contents of the tubes, and let stand for a minimum of 2 minutes but no longer than 10 minutes. Use a stopwatch or timer to make sure you perform the next step within the appropriate time frame.	☐	☐	______

Steps *(Continued)*	**Y**	**N**	**Number of Attempts**
11. Mix the contents of tubes again, then observe the degree of turbidity seen in each test tube and score as follows:			
NEG: No turbidity or cloudiness; urine remains clear	☐	☐	______
TRACE: Slight turbidity	☐	☐	______
1+: Turbidity with no precipitation (print on a page held behind tube is visible)	☐	☐	______
2+: Heavy turbidity with fine granulation	☐	☐	______
3+: Heavy turbidity with granulation and flakes	☐	☐	______
4+: Clumps of precipitated protein	☐	☐	______
The specimen may be matched against a McFarland standard to decrease the degree of subjective interpretation.	☐	☐	______
12. Clean work area, and dispose of all waste properly. Remove gown, gloves, and face shield. Wash your hands.	☐	☐	______

☐ **Pass** ☐ **Fail**

Comments

____

____

____

____

Procedure 28-10 Performing Diazo Tablet Test (Ictotest) for Bilirubin

NAME ______________________ **DATE/TIME** ______________

EVALUATED ______________________ **SCORE** ______________

Goal—To perform a diazo tablet test (Ictotest) for bilirubin.

Objectives/Conditions—When asked to perform a diazo tablet test (Ictotest) for bilirubin, the student will obtain appropriate supplies and equipment and correctly demonstrate how this test is performed.

Outcome—A diazo tablet test (Ictotest) for bilirubin is performed in accordance with the steps presented in the text.

Equipment and Supplies

Patient's labeled urine specimen
Octotest white mats
Clean paper towel
Transfer pipette
Stopwatch or timer

Steps

Steps	Y	N	Number of Attempts
1. Wash your hands.	☐	☐	______
2. Assemble the equipment.	☐	☐	______
3. Put on impervious gown, gloves, and face shield.	☐	☐	______
4. Verify that the names on the specimen container and the laboratory form are the same.	☐	☐	______
5. Place an Ictotest white mat on a clean, dry paper towel.	☐	☐	______
6. Using a clean transfer pipette, add 10 drops of the patient's urine to the center of the mat. (If the urine is red, it may be difficult to read the reaction properly. Pour a representative sample [aliquot] of the urine into a urine tube or test tube, and centrifuge as you would for preparing urine sediment. Use 10 drops of supernatant in this step.)	☐	☐	______
7. Shake a tablet into the bottle cap, and dispense onto the center of the mat. Do not touch the tablet with your hands.	☐	☐	______
8. Recap the bottle immediately.	☐	☐	______
9. Using a clean transfer pipette, place 1 drop of water on the tablet and wait 5 seconds.	☐	☐	______
10. Add another drop of water to the tablet so that the solution formed by the first drop runs onto the mat.	☐	☐	______
11. Within 60 seconds, observe for either a blue or purple color on the mat around the tablet. Either color indicates a positive result. Pink or red indicates a negative result.	☐	☐	______

Steps *(Continued)*	Y	N	Number of Attempts
12. Clean the work area, and dispose of waste properly. Remove gown, gloves, and face shield. Wash your hands.	☐	☐	______

☐ **Pass** ☐ **Fail**

Comments

____

____

____

____

Procedure 28-11 Preparing a Urine Sediment

NAME ______________________ **DATE/TIME** ______________

EVALUATED ______________________ **SCORE** ______________

Goal—To prepare a urine sediment.
Objectives/Conditions—When asked to prepare a urine sediment, the student will obtain appropriate equipment and supplies and correctly demonstrate the procedure.
Outcome—A urine sediment is prepared in accordance with the steps presented in the text.

Equipment and Supplies

Patient's labeled urine specimen
Urine centrifuge tubes
Transfer pipette
Centrifuge (1,500–2,000 rotations per minute)

Steps	Y	N	Number of Attempts
1. Wash your hands.	☐	☐	______
2. Assemble the equipment.	☐	☐	______
3. Put on impervious gown, gloves, and face shield.	☐	☐	______
4. Verify that the names on the specimen container and the laboratory form are the same.	☐	☐	______
5. Pour 10 to 15 mL of the patient's well-mixed urine into a labeled centrifuge tube (or a standardized system tube). Cap the tube with a plastic cap or parafilm.	☐	☐	______
6. Place the labeled urine tube in the centrifuge, and balance it with another tube (filled to the same level with water or another patient's urine).	☐	☐	______
7. Close the centrifuge cover and set it to spin at 1,500 RPM for 5 minutes.	☐	☐	______
8. When the centrifuge has stopped, remove the tubes. Make sure no tests are to be performed first on the supernatant. Remove the caps and pour off the supernatant, leaving a small portion of it (0.5–1.0 mL). Resuspend the sediment by flicking the tube with your finger or aspirating up and down with a transfer pipette, or follow manufacturer's directions for standardized system.	☐	☐	______
9. Properly care for and dispose of equipment and supplies. Clean the work area. Remove gown, gloves, and shield. Wash your hands.	☐	☐	______

☐ Pass ☐ Fail

Comments

____

____

____

____

Procedure 28-12 Performing a Microscopic Examination of Urine

NAME ______________________ **DATE/TIME** ______________

EVALUATED ______________________ **SCORE** ______________

Goal—To perform a microscopic examination of urine.

Objectives/Conditions—When asked to perform a microscopic examination of urine, the student will obtain appropriate equipment and supplies and correctly demonstrate this examination.

Outcome—A microscopic examination of urine is performed in accordance with the steps presented in the text.

Equipment and Supplies

Patient's labeled urine tube
Transfer pipette
Microscope
Lens cleaner
Lens paper
Glass slide
Coverslip
Standardized sediment slide (if applicable)

Steps	Y	N	Number of Attempts
1. Wash your hands.	☐	☐	______
2. Assemble the equipment.	☐	☐	______
3. Put on impervious gown, gloves, and face shield.	☐	☐	______
4. Verify that the names on the specimen container and the laboratory form are the same.	☐	☐	______
5. Using a spun urine specimen, make sure the sediment is well mixed with the remaining 1 mL of urine.	☐	☐	______
6. Using the transfer pipette, place 1 drop of the urine mixture onto a clean glass slide or into the chamber of the standardized slide.	☐	☐	______
7. Place a coverslip on the drop of urine if using the glass slide.	☐	☐	______
8. Place the slide on the microscopic stage between the holding clips. Using the 10× objective, focus until the sediment structures (eg, cells) become clear.	☐	☐	______
9. Scan the edges of the slide for casts, about 10 to 15 fields. If a cast is present, use the 40× objective to identify the type (waxy, granular, hyaline, white blood cells [WBC], red blood cells [RBC]). To report the amount of casts present, take the average seen on *low power, 10× objective*. Example: 0–1 hyaline casts/LPF. Record on the worksheet and lab form any casts observed.	☐	☐	______
10. Scan the slide using the 40× objective for about 10 to 15 fields. Average the number of RBC, WBC, and epithelial cells observed. Record on the worksheet and lab form.	☐	☐	______

Steps (Continued)	Y	N	Number of Attempts
11. Observe the presence of bacteria, mucus, crystals, sperm, and yeast using 40× objective for 10 fields. Use references located in the laboratory area to identify structures as needed. Average the number or amount observed, and record on the worksheet and lab form.	☐	☐	______
12. Report your observations as follows:			
Epithelial: Rare, few, moderate, many	☐	☐	______
Casts: Number per LPF	☐	☐	______
Mucus: Trace, 1+, 2+, 3+, 4+	☐	☐	______
WBCs: Lowest number and highest number seen in 10 fields per HPF (*Example: 0–5 WBC/HPF*)	☐	☐	______
RBCs: Lowest number and highest number seen in 10 fields per HPF (*Example: 2–10 RBC/HPF*)	☐	☐	______
Bacteria: Trace, 1+, 2+, 3+, 4+	☐	☐	______
Crystals, yeast, sperm: Few, moderate, many	☐	☐	______
(Note: 1+ = few in some fields; 2+ = few in all fields; 3+ = many in all fields; 4+ = too numerous to count [TNTC].)	☐	☐	______
13. Clean the work area and dispose of waste properly. Remove gown, gloves, and shield. Wash your hands.	☐	☐	______

☐ **Pass** ☐ **Fail**

Comments

____

____

____

____

29

Phlebotomy

COMPETENCY PRACTICE

Vocabulary Assessment

Matching

Match the definition in Part 1 with the correct term in Part 2.

PART 1

1. link arterioles to venules
2. bright red blood
3. dark red blood
4. vessel feels spongy like an elastic tube
5. anterior bend of forearm
6. spirals and ridges of finger prints
7. common capillary puncture sites

PART 2

a. _____ whorl
b. _____ venous blood
c. _____ capillaries
d. _____ arterial blood
e. _____ finger and heel
f. _____ antecubital
g. _____ vein

Definitions

Define the following terms.

1. antiseptic

____

____

____

2. cyanotic

____

____

____

3. edema

____

____

____

4. hemolysis

5. palmer

6. thromboplastin

7. venule

Critical Thinking

1. Describe behavior that the medical assistant can display that will gain a patient's trust and confidence as well as minimize anxiety and divert attention from any discomfort associated with phlebotomy.

2. Identify the sites for capillary blood collection in infants under 3 months and older infants. What measures can be used to enhance blood flow?

Case Studies

1. Dr. Adams has ordered a blood glucose, blood culture, and CBC on his patient, Miss Applegate. In what order would these specimens be drawn? Why?

2. Mrs. Jones is allergic to latex. Identify the signs and symptoms of latex allergy. What is the treatment for an allergic reaction to latex?

CHARTING EXERCISE

With regard to Case Study #1, write a narrative note describing your actions.

Document on the Patient's Chart:

- Date and time
- Notification of physician
- Patient complaints/concerns
- Patient education
- Your signature

Date/Time	Conditions/Lab Results Patient Communication

Basic Writing Activities

Skill Drills

1. List seven items (equipment and/or supplies) needed for obtaining a venous specimen.

____

____

____

2. Identify three sites each for the collection of capillary and venous blood specimens.

____

____

____

3. Immediately following a venous blood collection, the medical assistant should perform these two steps to care for the puncture site properly.

____

____

____

4. Describe the steps in preparation of the site for venipuncture and skin puncture.

____

____

____

Fill-in-the-Blanks

1. Venous blood is low in _______________.
2. OSHA guidelines require that _______________ be worn when performing phlebotomy procedures.
3. _______________ in a 1:10 solution is commonly used to wipe surfaces and clean up blood spills in the phlebotomy station.
4. The frosted end of a slide allows the medical assistant to _______________.
5. The most commonly used antiseptic for routine blood collection is _______________.
6. Microcollection tubes are used for hematocrit determinations on _______________ of blood.
7. When performing a phlebotomy, the bevel of the needle should always be turned _______________.

Innovative Activities

Label Design

Design a label to be placed on a patient's chart that denotes a latex allergy.

COMPETENCY EVALUATION CHECKLIST

Procedure 29-1 Obtaining a Blood Specimen From a Patient by Venipuncture

NAME ______________________ **DATE/TIME** ______________

EVALUATED ______________________ **SCORE** ______________

Goal—To obtain a blood specimen from a patient by venipuncture.

Objectives/Conditions—When given equipment and supplies listed in the text, the student will obtain a blood specimen from a patient by venipuncture.

Outcome—The student will obtain a blood specimen from a patient by venipuncture in accordance with the steps in the text.

Equipment and Supplies

Needle, syringe, and tube(s) or evacuated tubes
Tourniquet
Sterile gauze pads
Bandages
Needle and adaptor
Sharps container
70% alcohol pad or alternative antiseptic
Permanent marker or pen

Steps	Y	N	Number of Attempts
1. Check the requisition slip to determine the tests ordered and specimen requirements.	☐	☐	________
2. Wash your hands.	☐	☐	________
3. Assemble the equipment. Check the expiration date on the tubes.	☐	☐	________
4. Greet and identify the patient. Explain the procedure. Ask for and answer any questions.	☐	☐	________
5. If a fasting specimen is required, ask the patient the last time food was eaten.	☐	☐	________
6. Put on nonsterile latex or vinyl gloves.	☐	☐	________
7. Break the seal of the needle cover, and thread the sleeved needle into the adaptor, using the needle cover as a wrench. Tap the tubes that contain additives to ensure that the additive is dislodged from the stopper and wall of the tube. Insert the tube into the adaptor until the needle slightly enters the stopper. Do not push the top of the tube stopper beyond the indentation mark. If the tube retracts slightly, leave it in the retracted position. If using a syringe, tighten the needle on the hub and "breathe" the syringe.	☐	☐	________

Steps (Continued)	Y	N	Number of Attempts
8. Instruct the patient to sit with the arm well supported in a downward extended position if possible.	☐	☐	______
a. Apply the tourniquet around the patient's arm 3 to 4 inches above the elbow.	☐	☐	______
b. Apply the tourniquet snugly, but not too tightly.	☐	☐	______
c. Secure the tourniquet by using the half-bow.	☐	☐	______
d. Make sure the tails of the tourniquet extend upward to avoid contaminating the venipuncture site.	☐	☐	______
e. Ask the patient to close his or her hand into a fist, but not to pump the fist.	☐	☐	______
9. Select a vein by palpating. Use your gloved index finger to trace the path of the vein and judge its depth.	☐	☐	______
10. Release the tourniquet after palpating the vein if it has been left on for more than 1 minute.	☐	☐	______
11. Cleanse the venipuncture site with an alcohol pad starting in the center of puncture site and working outward in a circular motion. Allow the site to dry or dry the site with sterile gauze. Do not touch the area after cleansing.	☐	☐	______
12. If blood being drawn for culture will be used in diagnosing septic conditions, make sure the specimen is sterile. To do this, apply alcohol to the area for 2 full minutes. Then apply a 2% iodine solution in ever-widening circles. Never move the wipes back over areas that have been cleaned; use a new wipe for each sweep across the area. Allow the iodine to dry completely.	☐	☐	______
13. Reapply the tourniquet if it was removed after palpation.	☐	☐	______
14. Remove the needle cover. Hold the syringe or evacuated assembly in your dominant hand. Your thumb should be on top of the adaptor and your fingers underneath. Grasp the patient's arm with the nondominant hand while using your thumb to draw the skin taut over the site and anchor the vein about 1 to 2 inches below the puncture site.	☐	☐	______
15. With the bevel up, line up the needle with the vein at approximately 1/4 to 1/2 inch below the site where the vein is to be entered. At a 15- to 30-degree angle, rapidly and smoothly insert the needle through the skin.	☐	☐	______
16. Remove your nondominant hand, and slowly pull back the plunger of the syringe. Instead, you may place two fingers on the flanges of the adapter, and with the thumb, push the tube onto the needle inside the adapter. When blood flow begins in the tube or syringe, release the tourniquet and allow the patient to release the fist. Allow the syringe or tube(s) to fill to capacity. When blood flow ceases, remove the tube from the adapter by gripping the tube with your nondominant hand, and place your thumb against the flange during removal.	☐	☐	______

Steps (Continued)	Y	N	Number of Attempts
17. Gently pull out the tube. If the tube contains an additive, immediately invert it 5 to 10 times.	☐	☐	______
18. Steady the needle in the vein. To prevent discomfort, try not to pull up or press down on the needle while it is in the vein. Insert any other necessary tubes into adapter and allow to fill to capacity.	☐	☐	______
19. Remove the tube from the adapter before removing the needle from the arm. If the tourniquet has not been previously released, do so now.	☐	☐	______
a. Place a sterile gauze pad over the puncture site at the time of needle withdrawal. Do not apply any pressure to the site until the needle is completely removed.	☐	☐	______
b. After the needle is removed, apply pressure or have the patient apply direct pressure for 3 to 5 minutes. Do not bend the arm at the elbow.	☐	☐	______
20. Transfer the blood from a syringe into the proper order of draw tubes by inserting the needle through the stopper and allowing the vacuum to fill the tubes. Do not hold the tube when puncturing the stopper and filling the tube; place it in a tube rack and carefully insert the needle through the stopper. If the vacuum tubes contain an anticoagulant, they must be mixed immediately by gently inverting the tube 8 to 10 times. Do not shake the tube. Label the tubes with the proper information.	☐	☐	______
21. Check the puncture site for bleeding. Apply a bandage.	☐	☐	______
22. Properly care for or dispose of all equipment and supplies. Clean the work area. Remove gloves and wash your hands.	☐	☐	______
23. Test, transfer, or store the blood specimens according to the medical office policy.	☐	☐	______

☐ Pass ☐ Fail

Comments

____

____

____

____

Procedure 29-2 Obtaining a Blood Specimen From a Patient by Skin Puncture

NAME ______________________ **DATE/TIME** ______________

EVALUATED ______________________ **SCORE** ______________

Goal—To obtain a blood specimen from a patient by skin puncture.

Objectives/Conditions—When given equipment and supplies listed in the text, the student will obtain a blood specimen from a skin puncture.

Outcome—The student will obtain a blood specimen from a patient by skin puncture in accordance with the steps in the text.

Equipment and Supplies

Sterile disposable lancet or automated skin puncture device
70% alcohol or alternative antiseptic sterile gauze pads
Collection containers (Unopetted, capillary tubes)
Heel-warming device (if needed)

Steps	Y	N	Number of Attempts
1. Check the requisition slip to determine the tests ordered and specimen requirements.	☐	☐	______
2. Wash your hands.	☐	☐	______
3. Assemble the equipment.	☐	☐	______
4. Greet and identify the patient. Explain the procedure. Ask for and answer any questions.	☐	☐	______
5. Put on nonsterile latex or vinyl gloves.	☐	☐	______
6. Select the puncture site (the lateral portion of the tip of the middle or ring finger of the nondominant hand, lateral curved surface of the heel, or the great toe of an infant). The puncture should be made in the fleshy, central portion of the second or third finger, slightly to the side of center, and perpendicular to the grooves of the fingerprint. Perform heel puncture only on the plantar surface of the heel, medial to an imaginary line extending from the middle of the great toe to the heel, and lateral to an imaginary line drawn from between the fourth and fifth toes to the heel. Puncture should not exceed 2.4 mm in depth.	☐	☐	______
7. Make sure the site chosen is warm and not cyanotic or edematous. Gently massage the finger from the base to the tip or warm the site for 3 minutes with a warm washcloth or commercial heel warmer.	☐	☐	______
8. Grasp the finger firmly between your nondominant index finger and the thumb, or grasp the infant's heel firmly with the index finger wrapped around the foot and the thumb wrapped around the ankle. Cleanse the ball of the selected finger or heel with 70% isopropyl alcohol and wipe dry with a sterile gauze pad or allow to air dry.	☐	☐	______

Steps (Continued)	Y	N	Number of Attempts
9. Hold the patient's finger or heel firmly, and make a swift, deep puncture. Perform the puncture perpendicular to the whorls of the fingerprint or footprint in a recommended safe area.	☐	☐	______
10. Wipe away the first drop of blood with a sterile dry gauze.	☐	☐	______
11. Apply pressure toward the site, but do not "milk" or squeeze the site.	☐	☐	______
12. Collect the required specimen in the chosen containers or slides. Touch only the tip of the collection device to the drop of blood. Blood flow is encouraged if the puncture site is held in a downward, or dependent, angle and a gentle pressure is applied to the site. Cap microcollection tubes with the caps provided, and mix the additives by gently tilting or inverting the tubes 8 to 10 times.	☐	☐	______
13. When collection is complete, apply pressure to the site with a clean gauze until bleeding stops. Label the containers with the proper information. Do not apply bandages to skin punctures of infants under 2 years of age. Never release a patient until the the bleeding has stopped.	☐	☐	______
14. Properly care for or dispose of equipment and supplies. Clean the work area. Remove gloves and wash your hands.	☐	☐	______
15. Test, transfer, or store the blood specimen according to the medical office policy.	☐	☐	______

☐ **Pass** ☐ **Fail**

Comments

____

____

____

____

30

Hematology

COMPETENCY PRACTICE

Vocabulary Assessment

Matching

Match the definition in Part 1 with the correct term in Part 2.

PART 1

1. blood cell production
2. characteristics that are measured
3. hormone released by kidneys that influences red cell production
4. measurements of hemoglobin, hematocrit cell volume, and so forth
5. variation of cell size
6. variation of cell shape
7. anticoagulant

PART 2

a. _____ anisocytosis

b. _____ poikilocytosis

c. _____ parameters

d. _____ indices

e. _____ erythropoietin

f. _____ Coumadin

g. _____ hematopoiesis

Definitions

Define each of the following terms.

1. femtoliter

____

____

____

2. folate

____

____

____

3. hyperosmolarity

____

____

____

4. autolet

____

____

____

5. heparin

____

____

____

6. coumarin

____

____

____

7. hematocytometer

____

____

____

Critical Thinking

1. Explain the principle of automated cell counters.

____

____

____

2. Describe the purpose for performing an ESR.

____

____

____

Case Studies

1. Mr. Allen has been on heparin for 6 weeks as treatment for a blood clot in his lungs. Today he is visiting Dr. Jones's office for a check-up. You will be assisting Dr. Jones in obtaining a blood specimen to monitor Mr. Allen's progress. What test will Dr. Jones be using to monitor Mr. Allen's heparin therapy? What will the results of the test tell Dr. Jones?

____

____

____

2. Ms. Peters is being treated for anemia. She has a follow-up appointment with Dr. Smith today. Dr. Smith requests that a hemoglobin measurement be taken. When Dr. Smith leaves the room Ms. Peters asks you "What is a hemoglobin measurement, and what will the results mean?" She also requests patient education information on types of anemia, which your office has available. What can you tell Ms. Peters about this blood test?

____

____

____

CHARTING EXERCISE

Using the situation described in Case Study #2, write a narrative chart note describing your interaction with the patient, including obtaining a blood specimen and patient education.

Document on the Patient's Chart:

- Date and time
- Notification of physician
- Patient complaints/concerns
- Patient education
- Your signature

Date/Time	Conditions/Lab Results Patient Communication

Basic Writing Activities

Skill Drills

1. List seven parameters that are measured in a complete blood count (CBC).

____

____

____

2. List four conditions that can diminish leukocytes.

____

____

____

3. List five conditions that can increase leukocytes.

____

____

____

4. Identify the five white cell types that are examined in a WBC differential.

____

____

____

Fill-in-the-Blanks

1. The hematocrit is the percentage of red blood cells contained in ______________.
2. Platelets (______________), like other blood cells, are made in the bone marrow.
3. Coagulation tests measure the ability of whole blood to form a ______________.
4. An example of an agranulocyte white blood cell is a ______________.
5. ______________ is a complex substance found in blood and tissues that aids in the clotting process.

Innovative Activities

Labeling

Label the cell slide pictures with the type of cells represented in each slide.

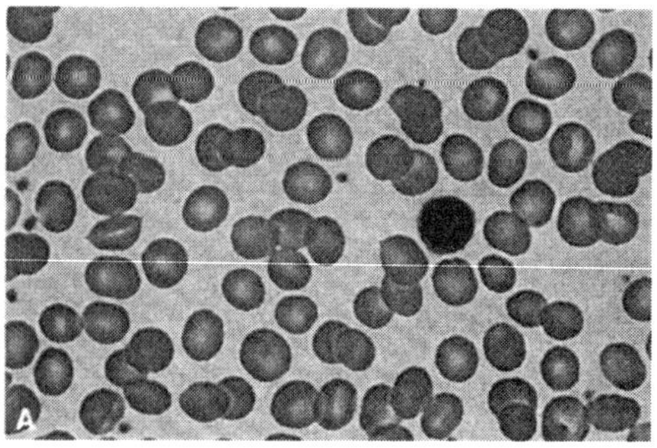

____

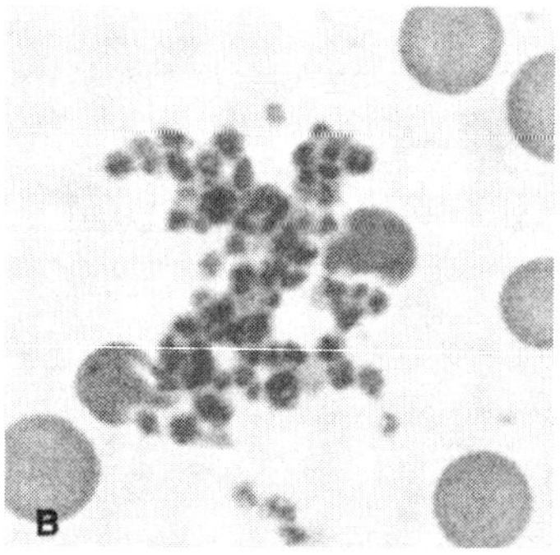

____

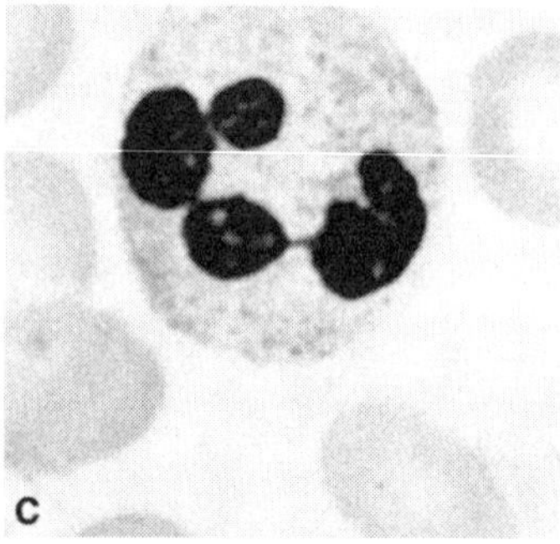

____

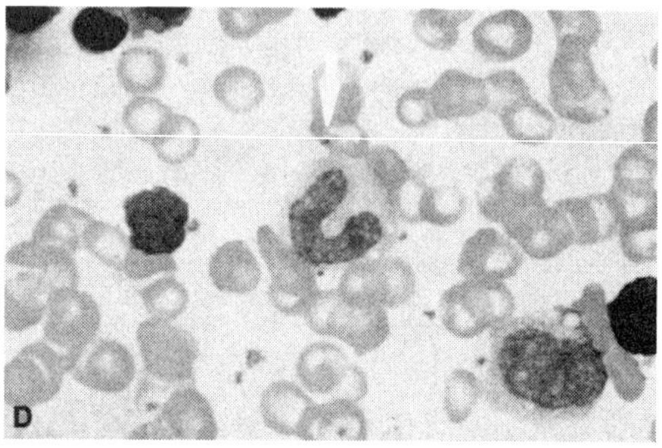

____

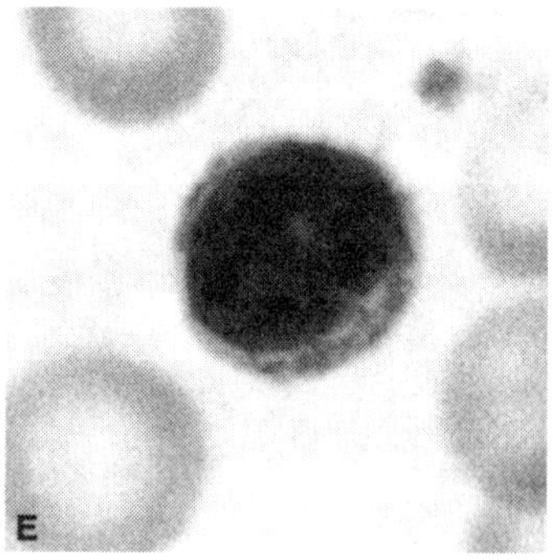

____

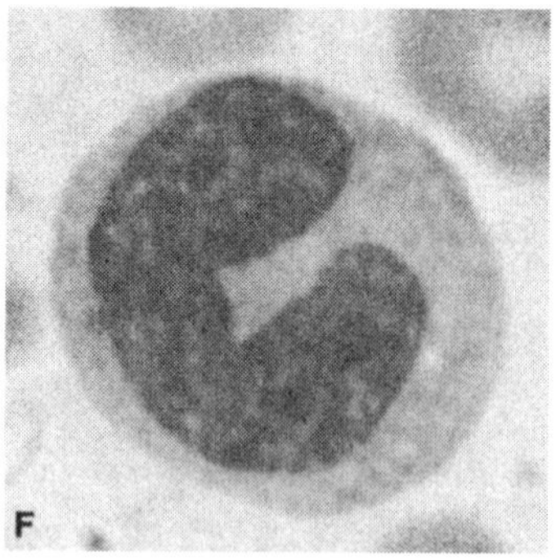

____

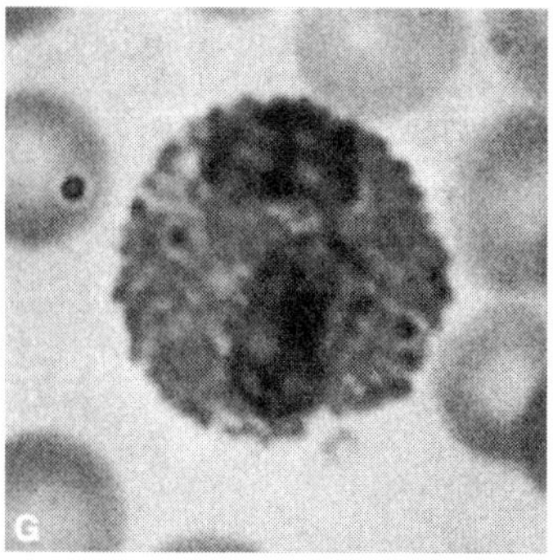

____

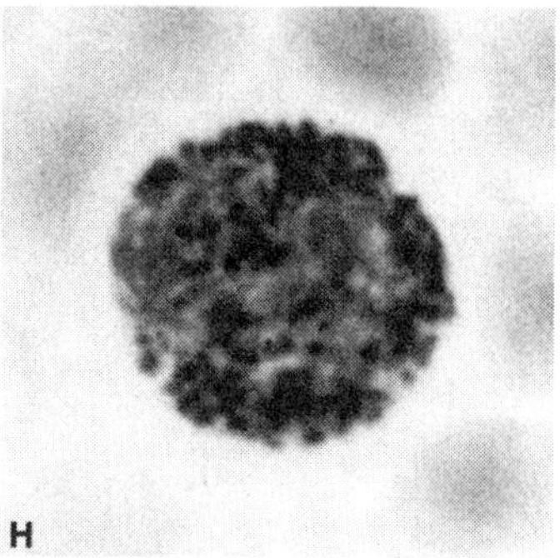

____

COMPETENCY EVALUATION CHECKLIST

Procedure 30-1 Performing a Manual WBC Count

NAME ______________________ **DATE/TIME** ______________

EVALUATED ______________________ **SCORE** ______________

Goal—To perform a manual WBC count.

Objectives/Conditions—When asked to perform a manual WBC count, the student will obtain appropriate equipment and supplies and correctly demonstrate how this lab test is to be performed.

Outcome—A manual WBC count is performed in accordance with the steps presented in the text.

Equipment and Supplies

Unopette system for WBC count
Neubauer hemacytometer
Cover glass
Gauze
Moist filter paper or moist cotton ball
Petri dish
Hand tally counter

Steps	Y	N	Number of Attempts
1. Wash your hands.	☐	☐	______
2. Assemble the equipment.	☐	☐	______
3. Using the shield on the capillary pipette, pierce the diaphragm in the neck of the reservoir, pushing the tip of the shield firmly through the diaphragm before removing it. Remove the shield from the capillary pipette using a twisting motion. Fill the pipette with free-flowing whole blood obtained through skin puncture or from a properly obtained, well-mixed EDTA (lavender top) tube specimen. (See Chap. 29, Phlebotomy, for the procedure for performing a skin puncture.)	☐	☐	______
4. If filling from a tube, place the tip of the Unopette just below the surface of the blood. Allow capillary action to fill the Unopette system completely.	☐	☐	______
5. Wipe off the pipette with gauze, being careful not to draw it across the tip.	☐	☐	______
6. Squeeze the reservoir gently to press out the air without expelling any of the specimen. Place your finger over the opening of the overflow chamber of the pipette.	☐	☐	______
7. Maintain the pressure on the reservoir and your finger position on the pipette, and insert the pipette into the reservoir.	☐	☐	______
8. Release the reservoir pressure. Then remove your finger from the pipette.	☐	☐	______
9. Gently press and release the reservoir several times, forcing the diluent into but not out of the overflow chamber.	☐	☐	______
10. Place your index finger over the opening of the overflow chamber, and gently invert or swirl the container several times. Remove your finger, and cover the opening with the pipette shield.	☐	☐	______

Steps (Continued)	Y	N	Number of Attempts
11. Label with the required patient information, and set the unit aside for 10 minutes.	☐	☐	____
12. At the proper interval, mix the contents again by gently swirling the assembly.	☐	☐	____
13. Remove the pipette from the Unopette reservoir, and replace it as a dropper assembly.	☐	☐	____
14. Invert the reservoir and gently squeeze the sides, discarding the first 3 to 4 drops.	☐	☐	____
15. Charge the hemacytometer by touching the tip of the assembly to the V-shaped loading area of the covered chamber. Control the flow gently, and do not overfill. Do not allow the specimen to flow into the H-shaped moats that surround the platform loading area.	☐	☐	____
16. Place the hemacytometer and the moistened filter paper or cotton ball in the Petri dish, and cover the entire assembly for 5 to 10 minutes.	☐	☐	____
17. Place the prepared hemacytometer on the microscope stage, and turn to the 100× magnification.	☐	☐	____
18. Using a zigzag counting pattern; starting at the top far left, count the top row left to right. At the end of the top row, drop to the second row, and count from right to left.	☐	☐	____
19. Using the tally counter, count all of the WBCs within the boundaries and those that touch the top and left borders. Do not count those that touch the bottom or right borders.	☐	☐	____
20. Record the number. Return the tally counter to 0, and move to the next square until all nine squares have been counted. If the numbers do not match by within 10%, the hemacytometer was improperly charged, and the test must be repeated. Count the opposite side of the hemacytometer.	☐	☐	____
21. Add the total from both sides of the hemacytometer and divide by 2. Add 10% to the averaged total.	☐	☐	____
22. Multiply this figure by 100.	☐	☐	____
23. Clean the hemacytometer and cover glass with 10% bleach solution, and wipe dry with lens paper.	☐	☐	____
24. Clean the work area. Remove your PPE, and wash your hands.	☐	☐	____

☐ **Pass** ☐ **Fail**

Comments

____

____

____

____

Procedure 30-2 Making a Peripheral Blood Smear

NAME ______________________________ **DATE/TIME** ______________

EVALUATED ______________________________ **SCORE** ______________

Goal—To make a peripheral blood smear.

Objectives/Conditions—When asked to make a peripheral blood smear, the student will obtain appropriate equipment and supplies and correctly make a peripheral blood smear.

Outcome—A peripheral blood smear is made in accordance with the steps presented in the text.

Equipment and Supplies

Clean glass slides with frosted ends
Transfer pipette
Whole blood
Pencil
Well-mixed patient specimen

Steps	Y	N	Number of Attempts
1. Wash your hands.	☐	☐	________
2. Assemble the equipment.	☐	☐	________
3. Greet and identify the patient. Explain the procedure. Ask for and answer any questions.	☐	☐	________
4. Put on gloves, impervious gown, and face shield.	☐	☐	________
5. Obtain an EDTA (lavender-top tube) blood specimen from the patient, following the steps for venipuncture described in Chap. 29, Phlebotomy.	☐	☐	________
6. Label the slide on the frosted area.	☐	☐	________
7. Place a drop of blood 1 cm from the frosted end of the slide.	☐	☐	________
8. Place the slide on a flat surface. With the thumb and forefinger of the right hand hold the second (spreader) slide against the surface of the first at a 30-degree angle. Draw the spreader slide back against the drop of blood until contact is established. (*Note:* The angle of the spreader slide may have to be greater than 30 degrees for larger or thinner drops of blood, and less than 30 degrees for smaller or thicker drops of blood.) Allow the blood to spread out under the edge, then push the spreader slide at a moderate speed toward the other end of the slide, keeping contact between the two slides at all times.	☐	☐	________
9. Allow the slide to air dry. (See the figures for examples of properly and improperly prepared smears.)	☐	☐	________

Steps (Continued)	Y	N	Number of Attempts
10. Properly care for or dispose of equipment and supplies. Clean the work area. Remove gloves, gown, and face shield, and wash your hands.	☐	☐	______

☐ Pass ☐ Fail

Comments

______

______

______

______

Procedure 30-3 Staining a Peripheral Blood Smear

NAME ______________________________ **DATE/TIME** _______________

EVALUATED ______________________________ **SCORE** __________

Goal—To stain a peripheral blood smear.

Objectives/Conditions—When asked to stain a peripheral blood smear, the student will obtain appropriate equipment and supplies and correctly demonstrate the staining of a peripheral blood smear.

Outcome—A peripheral blood smear is stained in accordance with the steps presented in the text.

Equipment and Supplies

Staining rack
Wright's stain
Giemsa stain
Prepared slide
Tweezers

Steps	Y	N	Number of Attempts
1. Wash your hands.	☐	☐	______
2. Assemble the equipment.	☐	☐	______
3. Put on gloves, impervious gown, and face shield.	☐	☐	______
4. Obtain a recently made, dried blood smear.	☐	☐	______
5. Place the slide on a stain rack blood side up.	☐	☐	______
6. Flood the slide with Wright's stain. Allow the stain to remain on the slide for 3 to 5 minutes or for the time specified by the manufacturer.	☐	☐	______
7. Using tweezers, tilt the slide so that the stain drains off. Apply equal amounts of Giemsa stain and water. A green sheen will appear on the surface. Allow the stain to remain on the slide for 5 minutes or the time specified by the manufacturer.	☐	☐	______
8. Holding the slide with tweezers, gently rinse the slide with water. Wipe off the back of the slide with gauze. Stand the slide upright and allow it to dry.	☐	☐	______
9. Properly care for or dispose of equipment and supplies. Clean the work area. Remove gloves, gown, and face shield, and wash your hands.	☐	☐	______

☐ **Pass** ☐ **Fail**

Comments

Procedure 30-4 Performing a WBC Differential

NAME ______________________ **DATE/TIME** ______________

EVALUATED ______________________ **SCORE** ______________

Goal—To perform a WBC differential.

Objectives/Conditions—When asked to perform a WBC differential, the student will obtain appropriate equipment and supplies and correctly perform a WBC differential.

Outcome—A WBC differential is performed in accordance with the steps presented in the text.

Equipment and Supplies

Stained peripheral blood smear
Microscope
Immersion oil
Paper
Recording tabulator

Steps	Y	N	Number of Attempts
1. Wash your hands.	☐	☐	______
2. Assemble the equipment.	☐	☐	______
3. Put on gloves.	☐	☐	______
4. Place the stained slide on the microscope. Focus on the feathered edge of the smear and scan to ensure an even distribution of cells and proper staining. Use the low-power objective.	☐	☐	______
5. Carefully turn the nosepiece to the high-power objective and bring the slide into focus using the fine adjustment.	☐	☐	______
6. Place a drop of oil on the slide, and rotate the oil immersion lens into place. Focus and begin to identify any leukocytes present.	☐	☐	______
7. Record on a tally sheet or tabulator the type of white cells found.	☐	☐	______
8. Move the stage so that the next field is in view. Identify any white cells in this field, and continue to the next field to identify all that are present until 100 white cells have been counted.	☐	☐	______
9. Calculate the number of each type of leukocyte as a percentage.	☐	☐	______
10. Properly care for or dispose of equipment and supplies. Clean the work area. Remove gloves, and wash your hands.	☐	☐	______

☐ **Pass** ☐ **Fail**

Comments

____

____

____

____

Procedure 30-5 Performing a Manual RBC Count

NAME ______________________ **DATE/TIME** ______________

EVALUATED ______________________ **SCORE** ______________

Goal—To perform a manual RBC count.

Objectives/Conditions—When asked to perform a manual RBC count, the student will obtain appropriate equipment and supplies and correctly demonstrate this lab procedure.

Outcome—A manual RBC count is performed in accordance with the steps presented in the text.

Equipment and Supplies

Unopette system for red cell count
Clean, lint-free hemacytometer
Cover glass
Gauze
Moist filter paper or moist cotton ball
Petri dish
Microscope
Hand tally counter

Steps	Y	N	Number of Attempts
1–16. Follow steps 1–16 listed in Procedure 30-1: Performing a Manual White Blood Cell Count.	☐	☐	______
17. Place the hemacytometer on the microscope stage so that the ruled area can be surveyed with the low-power objective. Focus the microscope, then progress to the 400× magnification to count the RBCs.	☐	☐	______
18. Count the RBCs in the four corner squares and the center square following the zigzag pattern described in Procedure 30-1. Starting at the top far left, count the top row left to right. At the end of the top row, drop to the second row, and count from right to left. Continue this pattern until all of the rows are counted. Count cells touching the upper and left side, but do not count those on the lower and right side.	☐	☐	______
19. Tally the count and record the number. Return the counter to 0 and count the next grid. Count the opposite side of the hemacytometer.	☐	☐	______
20. The count within the squares should not vary by more than 20 cells. If the variance is greater, the test must be repeated.	☐	☐	______
21. Average the two sides, and multiply the result by 10,000.	☐	☐	______

Steps (Continued)	Y	N	Number of Attempts
22. Clean the hemacytometer and cover glass with 10% bleach, and wipe dry with lens paper. Dispose of or care for any other equipment and supplies appropriately. Clean the work area. Remove gloves and gown, and wash your hands.	☐	☐	______

☐ **Pass** ☐ **Fail**

Comments

____

____

____

____

Procedure 30-6 Performing a Hemoglobin Determination

NAME ____________________ **DATE/TIME** ____________

EVALUATED ____________________ **SCORE** ____________

Goal—To perform a hemoglobin determination.

Objectives/Conditions—When asked to perform a hemoglobin determination, the student will obtain appropriate equipment and supplies and correctly demonstrate this lab procedure.

Outcome—A hemoglobin determination is performed in accordance with the steps presented in the text.

Equipment and Supplies

Hemoglobinometer
Applicator sticks
Whole blood

Steps	Y	N	Number of Attempts
1. Wash your hands.	☐	☐	______
2. Assemble the necessary equipment.	☐	☐	______
3. Put on gloves, gown, and face shield.	☐	☐	______
4. Obtain an EDTA (lavender-top tube) blood specimen from the patient, following the steps for capillary puncture described in Chap. 29, Phlebotomy.	☐	☐	______
5. Place a drop of well-mixed whole blood (obtained by skin puncture) on the glass chamber of the hemoglobinometer. Place the coverslip into the holding clip over the chamber and slide it into the holding clip.	☐	☐	______
6. At one of the open edges, push the applicator stick into the chamber. Gently move the stick around until the specimen no longer appears cloudy.	☐	☐	______
7. Slide the chamber into the hemoglobinometer. Remove the face shield.	☐	☐	______
8. With your left hand, hold the meter and press the light button. View the field through the eyepiece. With your right hand, move the dial until both of the right and left sides match each other in color intensity. Note the hemoglobin level indicated on the dial.	☐	☐	______
9. Clean the chamber and work area with 10% bleach solution. Dispose of equipment and supplies appropriately. Remove gloves and gown, and wash your hands.	☐	☐	______

☐ Pass ☐ Fail

Comments

____

____

____

____

Procedure 30-7 Performing a Microhematocrit Determination

NAME ______________________ **DATE/TIME** ______________

EVALUATED ______________________ **SCORE** ______________

Goal—To perform a microhematocrit determination.

Objectives/Conditions—When asked to perform a microhematocrit determination, the student will obtain appropriate equipment and supplies and correctly demonstrate this lab procedure.

Outcome—A microhematocrit determination is performed in accordance with the steps presented in the text.

Equipment and Supplies

Microcollection tubes
Sealing clay
Microhematocrit centrifuge
Microhematocrit reading device

Steps	Y	N	Number of Attempts
1. Wash your hands.	☐	☐	________
2. Assemble the equipment.	☐	☐	________
3. Put on gloves, gown, and face shield.	☐	☐	________
4. Draw blood into the capillary tube by one of two methods: (1) directly from a capillary puncture where the tip of the capillary tube is touched to the blood at the wound and allowed to fill 3/4 of the tube or to the indicated mark (see Chap. 29, Phlebotomy); or (2) from a well mixed anticoagulated (EDTA) tube of whole blood where, again, the tip is touched to the blood and allowed to fill 3/4 of the tube. Place the forefinger over the top of the tube, wipe excess blood off the sides, and push the bottom into the sealing clay. Draw a second specimen in the same manner.	☐	☐	________
5. Place the tubes in the radial grooves of the microhematocrit centrifuge opposite each other. Place the cover on top of the grooved area, and tighten by turning the knob clockwise. Close the lid. Spin for 5 minutes or as directed by the manufacturer.	☐	☐	________
6. Remove the tubes from the centrifuge and read the results from the reading device available (instructions are printed on the device). (The accompanying figure shows two methods for determining microhematocrit values.) Results should match within 5% of each other. Take the average and report as a percentage. (*Note:* Some microhematocrit centrifuges have the scale printed within the machine at the radial grooves.)	☐	☐	________

Steps (Continued)	Y	N	Number of Attempts
7. Dispose of the microhematocrit tubes in a biohazard container. Properly care for or dispose of other equipment and supplies. Clean the work area. Remove gloves, gown, and face shield, and wash your hands.	☐	☐	______

☐ Pass ☐ Fail

Comments

____

____

____

____

Procedure 30-8 Performing a Wintrobe ESR

NAME ______________________ **DATE/TIME** ______________

EVALUATED ______________________ **SCORE** ______________

Goal—To perform a Wintrobe ESR.
Objectives/Conditions—When asked to perform a Wintrobe ESR, the student will obtain appropriate equipment and supplies and correctly demonstrate this lab procedure.
Outcome—A Wintrobe ESR is performed in accordance with the steps presented in the text.

Equipment and Supplies

Anticoagulation tube
Wintrobe tube
Transfer pipette
Timer

Steps	Y	N	Number of Attempts
1. Wash your hands.	☐	☐	______
2. Assemble the necessary equipment.	☐	☐	______
3. Put on gloves, impervious gown, and face shield.	☐	☐	______
4. Draw blood (see Chap. 29, Phlebotomy) into an EDTA lavender-stoppered anticoagulation tube.	☐	☐	______
5. Fill a graduated Wintrobe tube to the 0 mark with the well mixed whole (EDTA) blood using the provided transfer pipette. Be sure to eliminate any trapped bubbles and fill exactly to the 0 line.	☐	☐	______
6. Place the tube in a holder that will allow the tube to remain in a vertical position.	☐	☐	______
7. Wait exactly 1 hour; use a timer for accuracy. Keep the tube straight upright and undisturbed during the hour.	☐	☐	______
8. Record the level of the top of the red blood cells after 1 hour. Normal results for men are 0–10 mL/h; for women, 0–15 mL/h.	☐	☐	______
9. Properly care for or dispose of equipment and supplies. Clean the work area. Remove gloves, gown, and face shield. Wash your hands.	☐	☐	______

☐ **Pass** ☐ **Fail**

Comments

____
____
____
____

Procedure 30-9 Determining Bleeding Time

NAME ______________________ **DATE/TIME** ______________

EVALUATED ______________________ **SCORE** ______________

Goal—To determine bleeding time.

Objectives/Conditions—When asked to determine bleeding time, the student will obtain appropriate equipment and supplies and correctly demonstrate this lab procedure.

Outcome—Bleeding time is determined in accordance with the steps presented in the text.

Equipment and Supplies

Blood pressure cuff
Autolet device
Alcohol or antiseptic wipe
Filter paper
Butterfly bandage
Stopwatch

Steps	Y	N	Number of Attempts
1. Wash your hands.	☐	☐	______
2. Assemble the equipment.	☐	☐	______
3. Greet and identify the patient. Explain the procedure. Ask for and answer any questions.	☐	☐	______
4. Put on gloves, impervious gown, and face shield.	☐	☐	______
5. Position the patient so that the arm is extended in a manner that is both comfortable and stable.	☐	☐	______
6. Have the patient turn the palm upward so that the inner aspect of the arm is exposed. Select a site several inches below the antecubital area. The area should be free of lesions and with no visible veins. Clean the site with alcohol or antiseptic wipe.	☐	☐	______
7. Apply the pressure cuff and set it at 40 mm Hg for the length of the test. Adjust it as needed throughout the test to maintain the pressure.	☐	☐	______
8. Twist the tear-away tab on the Autolet. Make an incision 1 mm in depth on the cleaned skin surface by placing the Autolet bleeding time device on the site and pressing the trigger button on the side. This will spring the blade to make the incision. At the same time, start the stop watch.	☐	☐	______
9. At 30-second intervals, bring the filter paper near the edge of the wound to draw off some of the accumulating blood. Avoid touching the wound with the filter paper.	☐	☐	______
10. The test is complete when the blood flow stops completely. Stop the watch when the blood no longer stains the filter paper; note the time to the nearest 30 seconds.	☐	☐	______
11. Apply a butterfly bandage across the wound to keep it sealed and cover the site with a waterproof bandage. Instruct the patient to keep the site dry and not to remove the bandage for a minimum of 24 hours.	☐	☐	______

Steps (Continued)	Y	N	Number of Attempts
12. Properly care for or dispose of all equipment and supplies. Clean the work area. Remove gloves, gown, and face shield, and wash your hands.	☐	☐	______

☐ **Pass** ☐ **Fail**

Comments

____

____

____

____

31

Serology and Immunohematology

COMPETENCY PRACTICE

Vocabulary Assessment

Matching

Match the definition in Part 1 with the correct term in Part 2.

PART 1

1. foreign substance to body
2. proteins produced by body
3. antibody that has particular attraction for its antigen
4. binding of antigens and antibodies
5. produced when whole blood is allowed to clot
6. study of antigens and antibodies

PART 2

a. _____ serology

b. _____ serum

c. _____ antigen

d. _____ antibodies

e. _____ sensitivity

f. _____ agglutination

Definitions

Define each of the following terms.

1. conjugate

____

____

____

2. hemolysis

____

____

____

3. specificity

____

____

____

4. substrate

____

____

____

Critical Thinking

1. Explain how syphilis is transmitted and by what bacteria, the most common age range of occurrence, and how it is treated.

____

____

____

2. The rubella virus causes a disease also known as German or 3-day measles. Explain when measles commonly occur and whether there is any protection against the disease. Describe symptoms and the effect on a fetus of less than 3 months' gestation.

____

____

____

Case Studies

1. Mrs. Jones is scheduled for an angioplasty in 6 weeks. Her physician would like a CBC drawn as well as four units of blood available during the surgery in case it is needed. Describe the three types of donated blood.

____

____

____

2. Mrs. Maxwell brings her 15-year-old son Jason in to see Dr. Stone. Jason complains of a sore throat, swollen lymph nodes, and feeling tired. Dr. Stone asks you to obtain a blood specimen from Jason and to send the specimen to the lab. Dr. Stone is trying to determine whether Jason has infectious mononucleosis. Jason tells you that he has heard of "mono" before and asks you to tell him more about it. What can you tell this patient?

____

____

____

CHARTING EXERCISE

Using the situation described in Case Study #2, write a narrative chart note describing your interaction with the patient.

Document on the Patient's Chart:

- Date and time
- Notification of physician
- Patient complaints/concerns
- Patient education
- Your signature

Date/Time	Conditions/Lab Results Patient Communication

Basic Writing Activities

Skill Drills

1. List five indications for serologic testing.

____

____

____

2. List the four areas to address to ensure quality assurance and quality control in serological testing.

____

____

____

3. List six serological tests most commonly encountered in the medical office.

____

____

____

4. List the three most common methods of enhancing the antigen–antibody reaction for testing purposes.

____

____

____

Fill-in-the-Blanks

1. Many serology tests require a ______________ specimen.
2. Rheumatoid arthritis is an autoimmune progressive inflammatory disease of the ______________.
3. Rapid plasma reagin (RPR) is a screening test for ______________.
4. The test for pregnancy is based on the detection of the hormone ______________ ______________.
5. Generally, blood donors must weigh more than ______________ pounds.

Innovative Activities

Create an educational brochure, appropriate to an obstetrician's office, regarding expectant mothers and RhoGAM.

COMPETENCY EVALUATION CHECKLIST

Procedure 31-1 Performing a Mononucleosis Test

NAME ______________________ **DATE/TIME** ______________

EVALUATED ______________________ **SCORE** ______________

Goal—To perform a mononucleosis test.

Objectives/Conditions—When asked to perform a mononucleosis test, the student will obtain appropriate equipment and supplies and correctly demonstrate the methods and techniques required for performing this test.

Outcome—A mononucleosis test is performed in accordance with the steps presented in the text.

Equipment and Supplies

Patient's labeled specimen (whole blood, plasma, or serum depending on the kit)
Mononucleosis kit (slide or card, controls, reagens, capillary tubes, bulb and stirrers)
Stopwatch or timer
Saline, test tubes, pipettes (if titration is required)

Steps	Y	N	Number of Attempts
1. Wash your hands.	☐	☐	______
2. Verify that the names on the specimen container and the laboratory form are the same.	☐	☐	______
3. Assemble the equipment, and ensure that the materials in the kit are at room temperature before beginning the procedure.	☐	☐	______
4. Label the slide or card (depending on the type of kit used) with the patient's name, positive control, and negative control. One circle or space is provided per patient and control.	☐	☐	______
5. Place the rubber bulb on the capillary tube, and aspirate the patient's specimen up to the marked line. Dispense the sample in the middle of the circle labeled with the patient's name. Avoid air bubbles to ensure accurate results.	☐	☐	______
6. Gently mix the positive control. Using the capillary tube, aspirate the positive control up to the marked line. Dispense the control in the middle of the circle labeled "negative control." Avoid air bubbles.	☐	☐	______
7. Mix the latex reagent, and add 1 drop to each circle or space (patient sample, positive control, negative control). Avoid splashing the reagents, which can result in cross-contamination and incorrect results.	☐	☐	______
8. Using a clean stirrer for each test, mix the reagent with the patient sample and controls. Mix only one circle at a time, keeping within each circle. Going outside of the circle may lead to cross-contamination and incorrect results.	☐	☐	______
9. Gently rock the slide for 2 minutes, and observe for agglutination (clumping). Testing time may vary if using a disposable card.	☐	☐	______

Steps (Continued)	**Y**	**N**	**Number of Attempts**
10. Verify the results of the controls before documenting the patient's results. Log controls and patient information on the worksheet.	☐	☐	______
11. Read the kit's instructions if titration is required.	☐	☐	______
12. Clean the work area and dispose of waste properly. Wash the slide thoroughly with bleach and rinse with water before using again. Remove gown, gloves and shield. Wash your hands.	☐	☐	______

☐ **Pass** ☐ **Fail**

Comments

____

____

____

____

Procedure 31-2 Performing an HCG Pregnancy Test

NAME ____________________ **DATE/TIME** ____________

EVALUATED ____________________ **SCORE** ____________

Goal—To perform an HCG pregnancy test.

Objectives/Conditions—When asked to perform an HCG pregnancy test, the student will obtain appropriate equipment and supplies and correctly demonstrate the methods and techniques required for performing this test.

Outcome—An HCG pregnancy test is performed in accordance with the steps presented in the text.

Equipment and Supplies

Patient's labeled specimen (plasma, serum, or urine depending on the kit)
HCG pregnancy kit (test pack and transfer pipettes; kit contents will vary by manufacturer)
HCG positive and negative control (different controls may be needed when testing urine)
Timer

Steps	Y	N	Number of Attempts
1. Wash your hands.	☐	☐	________
2. Assemble the equipment.	☐	☐	________
3. Verify that the names on the specimen container and the laboratory form are the same.	☐	☐	________
4. Label the test pack (depending on type of kit) with the patient's name, positive control, and negative control. Use one test pack per patient and control.	☐	☐	________
5. Note in the patient's information and in the control log if you are using urine, plasma, or serum for testing. Be sure that the kit and controls are at room temperature for accurate testing.	☐	☐	________
6. Aspirate the patient's specimen using the transfer pipette and place three drops (180 μL) on the sample well of the test pack labeled with the patient's name.	☐	☐	________
7. Aspirate the positive control using the transfer pipette and place three drops (180 μL) on the sample well of the test pack labeled "positive control." Avoid splashing to eliminate cross-contamination.	☐	☐	________
8. Aspirate the negative control using the transfer pipette, and place three drops (180 μL) on the sample well of the test pack labeled "negative control." Avoid splashing to eliminate cross-contamination.	☐	☐	________
9. Report the results when the "End of Assay Window" is red. This will take approximately 7 minutes for serum samples and 4 minutes for urine samples. Check to verify controls before reporting the results. Repeat the test if the "End of Assay Window" does not appear and if the controls do not work.	☐	☐	________

Steps (Continued)	Y	N	Number of Attempts
10. Record controls and patient information on the worksheet and log form.	☐	☐	____________
11. Clean the work area and dispose of waste properly. Remove gown, gloves, and shield. Wash your hands.	☐	☐	____________

☐ **Pass** ☐ **Fail**

Comments

____

____

____

____

Procedure 31-3 Performing Group A Rapid Strep Test

NAME ______________________ **DATE/TIME** ______________

EVALUATED ______________________ **SCORE** ______________

Goal—To perform a group A rapid strep test.

Objectives/Conditions—When asked to perform a group A rapid strep test, the student will obtain appropriate equipment and supplies and correctly demonstrate how this test is to be performed.

Outcome—A group A rapid strep test is performed in accordance with the steps presented in the text.

Equipment and Supplies

Patient's labeled throat culture (use a culturette with two swabs provided)
Group A strep kit (controls may be included, depending on the kit)
Timer
Beta strep agar
Bacitracin disks
Note: Beta strep agar and bacitracin need to come to room temperature before being used.

Steps	Y	N	Number of Attempts
1. Wash your hands.	☐	☐	________
2. Verify that the names on the specimen container and the laboratory form are the same.	☐	☐	________
3. Label one extraction tube with the patient's name, another with the positive control, and one with the negative control.	☐	☐	________
4. Follow the directions for the kit. Add the appropriate reagents and drops to each of the extraction tubes. Avoid splashing, and use the correct number of drops.	☐	☐	________
5. Insert the patient's swab (one of the two swabs present) into the labeled extraction tube. If only one culture swab was submitted, first swab a beta strep agar plate, then use the swab for the rapid strep test.	☐	☐	________
6. Add the appropriate controls to each of the labeled extraction tubes.	☐	☐	________
7. Set the timer for the appropriate time to ensure testing accuracy.	☐	☐	________
8. Add the appropriate reagent and drops to each of the extraction tubes.	☐	☐	________
9. Use the swab to mix the reagents. Then press out any excess fluid remaining on the swab by placing your fingers on the outside of the extraction tube while pinching the swab against the inside of the tube.	☐	☐	________
10. Add three drops from the well mixed extraction tube to the sample window of the strep A test unit labeled with the patient's name. Do the same for each control.	☐	☐	________
11. Set the timer for the appropriate time.	☐	☐	________

Steps (Continued)	Y	N	Number of Attempts
12. Be aware that a positive result appears as a line in the result window within 5 minutes. An internal control is present in the strep A test unit; if a line appears in the control window, the test is valid.	☐	☐	______
13. Read a negative result at exactly 5 minutes to avoid a false-negative.	☐	☐	______
14. Verify results of the controls before recording test results. Log the controls and the patient information on the worksheet.	☐	☐	______
15. Note that depending on laboratory protocol, you may need to culture all negative rapid strep screens onto beta strep agar. A bacitracin disk may be added to the first quadrant while setting up or after 24 hours if a beta hemolytic colony appears. A culture is more sensitive than a rapid immunoassay test.	☐	☐	______
16. Clean the work area and dispose of waste properly. Remove gown, gloves, and shield. Wash your hands.	☐	☐	______

☐ **Pass** ☐ **Fail**

Comments

____

____

____

____

32

Clinical Chemistry

COMPETENCY PRACTICE

Vocabulary Assessment

Matching

Match the definition in Part 1 with the correct term in Part 2.

PART 1

1. sodium level too high
2. potassium level too high
3. magnesium level too high
4. test of choice for diabetic glucose testing
5. main ingredient of adipose tissue
6. calcium level too high
7. condition caused by high uric acid levels in joints

PART 2

a. _____ hyperkalemia
b. _____ hemoglobin A1-C
c. _____ triglycerides
d. _____ hypermagnesemia
e. _____ gout
f. _____ hypernatremia
g. _____ hypercalcemia

Definitions

Define each of the following terms.

1. catalyzes

____

____

____

2. challenge

____

____

____

3. nitrogenous

____

____

____

4. quantification

5. screening

Critical Thinking

1. Explain how the pancreas functions in both the endocrine and exocrine systems.

2. Describe the role that creatine plays in delivering energy to the cells of the body.

Case Studies

1. Wanda Nagle, aged 54, fasted for 14 hours prior to having a cholesterol test. You perform the test in the office lab on 11/6/00, at 9:00 a.m. As she is leaving the office she asks you what the ideal cholesterol range is and what the difference is between low-density and high-density lipoproteins. The physician will see this patient next week and give her the test results at that time.

2. Mr. Jeffers, aged 57, fasted for 14 hours prior to having a fasting blood sugar test. You perform the test in the office lab on 3/12/00, at 9:00 a.m. As he is leaving, he asks you what the normal range for an FBS is. He tells you that even though he has a family history of diabetes mellitus he really does not know much about the disease. How can you educate this patient on diabetes mellitus, including normal ranges for FBS?

CHARTING EXERCISE

Using the situation described in Case Study #1, write a narrative chart note describing your interaction with the patient.

Document on the Patient's Chart:

- Date and time
- Notification of physician
- Patient complaints/concerns
- Patient education
- Your signature

Date/Time	Conditions/Lab Results Patient Communication

Basic Writing Activities

Skill Drills

1. List six common tests performed in determining liver function and give the normal values of each.

____

____

____

2. List seven electrolytes that are measured when assessing renal functionality. Identify the chemical symbol for each one.

____

____

____

3. List and describe four frequently ordered glucose tests.

____

____

____

Fill-in-the-Blanks

1. _______________ is the major protein in the blood.
2. Creatine kinase is found almost exclusively in skeletal muscle and _______________.
3. Specimens for blood gases are usually drawn from an _______________
4. In pancreatitis, _______________ is markedly increased.
5. Hypoglycemia is a syndrome characterized by FBS levels below _______________ mg/dL, and a variety of symptoms.

Innovative Activities

Create a patient education brochure titled *Risk Factors for Premature Atherosclerosis and Coronary Heart Disease.*

COMPETENCY EVALUATION CHECKLIST

Procedure 32-1 Determining Blood Glucose Using the Glucometer

NAME ______________________ **DATE/TIME** ______________

EVALUATED ______________________ **SCORE** ______________

Goal—To determine blood glucose using a glucometer.

Objectives/Conditions—When asked to determine blood glucose using a glucometer, the student will obtain appropriate equipment and supplies and correctly demonstrate how to perform this test.

Outcomes—Blood glucose is determined, using a glucometer, in accordance with the steps presented in the text.

Equipment and Supplies

Glucometer (or glucose meter of the physician's choice)
Glucose reagent stripe
Lancet
Alcohol pad
Sterile gauze
Paper towel

Steps	Y	N	Number of Attempts
1. Wash your hands.	☐	☐	______
2. Assemble the equipment and supplies.	☐	☐	______
3. Put on gloves before removing reagent strip.	☐	☐	______
4. Turn the glucometer on, and ensure that it is calibrated. The digits 888 appear on the display screen followed by the code of the strips being used.	☐	☐	______
5. Remove one reagent strip, lay it on the paper towel, and recap the container.	☐	☐	______
6. Greet and identify the patient. Explain the procedure. Ask for and answer any questions.	☐	☐	______
7. Have the patient wash his or her hands.	☐	☐	______
8. Cleanse the selected puncture site (finger) with alcohol.	☐	☐	______
9. Puncture the site with a lancet, following the steps described in Chap. 29, Phlebotomy. Wipe away the first drop of blood.	☐	☐	______
10. Turn the patient's hand palm down and gently squeeze the finger to form a large drop of blood.	☐	☐	______
11. Bring the reagent strip up to the finger and touch the pad to the blood. Do not touch the finger. Completely cover the pad with blood.	☐	☐	______
12. Immediately press the TIME button. The glucometer counts up to 60 seconds. (Meanwhile, apply pressure to the puncture wound with gauze.) At the end of 60 seconds, firmly wipe the blood off with a clean gauze. The glucometer continues to count for another 60 seconds. During this time, insert the reagent strip into the chamber with the pad side down.	☐	☐	______

Steps (Continued)	Y	N	Number of Attempts
13. Be aware that at 120 seconds, the glucometer reads the reaction strip and displays the result on the screen in mg/dL. If the glucose level is higher or lower than expected, refer to the troubleshooting guide provided by the manufacturer.	☐	☐	______
14. Properly care for or dispose of equipment and supplies. Clean the work area. Remove gloves, and wash your hands.	☐	☐	______

☐ Pass ☐ Fail

Comments

____

____

____

____

Procedure 32-2 Glucose Tolerance Test (GTT)

NAME ______________________ **DATE/TIME** ______________

EVALUATED ______________________ **SCORE** ______________

Goal—To perform a glucose tolerance test.

Objectives/Conditions—When asked to perform a glucose tolerance test, the student will obtain appropriate equipment and supplies and correctly demonstrate this test.

Outcomes—A glucose tolerance test is performed in accordance with the steps presented in the text.

Equipment and Supplies

Calibrated amount of glucose per the physician's order
Phlebotomy equipment
Glucose test strips
Glucose meter equipment
Alcohol wipes
Stopwatch

Steps	Y	N	Number of Attempts
1. Wash your hands.	☐	☐	______
2. Assemble the equipment and supplies.	☐	☐	______
3. Greet and identify the patient. Explain the procedure. Ask for and answer any questions.	☐	☐	______
4. Obtain a fasting glucose (FBS) specimen (red top) from the patient using the steps as outlined in the venipuncture procedure (see Chap. 29, Phlebotomy). It is recommended that laboratories test the blood sample before the glucose drink is administered; if the FBS exceeds a certain reading (eg, greater than 140 mg/dL), do not perform the GTT. Notify the physician.	☐	☐	______
5. Give the glucose drink to the patient to consume within a 5-minute period. Note the time the patient finishes the drink; this is the "START" of the test.	☐	☐	______
6. Exactly 30 minutes after the patient has finished the glucose drink, obtain another blood specimen. Label the specimen with the patient's name and time of collection.	☐	☐	______
7. Exactly 1 hour after the glucose drink, repeat step 7.	☐	☐	______
8. Exactly 2 hours after the glucose drink, repeat step 7.	☐	☐	______
9. Exactly 3 hours after the glucose drink, repeat step 7. Unless a GTT of longer than 3 hours has been requested, the testing is complete at this time. (For a longer GTT, continue specimen collection in the same manner for as many additional hours as required.)	☐	☐	______

Steps (Continued)	Y	N	Number of Attempts
10. If the specimens are to be tested by an outside laboratory, package as required, and arrange for transportation.	☐	☐	________
11. Properly care for or dispose of equipment and supplies. Clean the work area. Remove gloves and gown, and wash your hands.	☐	☐	________

☐ Pass ☐ Fail

Comments

____

____

____

____

Answer Key

CHAPTER 1

Vocabulary

Matching

1. d	3. e	5. a	7. c
2. g	4. f	6. b	

Spelling Applications

1. centigrade
2. Occupational Safety and Health Administration
3. disease
4. asepsis
5. normal flora
6. surgical asepsis

Case Studies

1. Gloves are used to protect both the patient and the medical assistant. The medical assistant does not want to introduce any pathogens into the open wound on Mrs. Garcia's hand. Conversely, the medical assistant does not want to be exposed to any bloodborne pathogens from Mrs. Garcia. To reduce the spread of pathogens via blood and body fluids, OSHA guidelines require the use of personal protective equipment (PPE) of which gloves are one type. In this particular situation, the use of gloves will prevent the spread of pathogens between the medical assistant and patient as well as to other individuals the medical assistant may come in contact with.

   Directions for infection control at home when caring for the wound: Mrs. Garcia should be instructed to wash her hands before and after changing the dressing. If sterile dressings are to be applied to the wound, Mrs. Garcia should be instructed on proper technique. And finally, Mrs. Garcia should be instructed on the disposal of wound dressings.
2. Various types of PPE (personal protective equipment):

gloves
mask
goggles
face shield
impervious gown

Three situations that would require the use of PPE:

1. Administration of IM injections: gloves
2. Assisting with the irrigation of a wound: gloves, face shield, impervious gown
3. Performing laboratory procedures: gloves, goggles, impervious gown

Charting Exercise

5/7/99 9:00 a.m.
Wound care reviewed with patient, including handwashing and dressing application.

S. Smith, MA

Fill-in-the-Blank

1. CDC (Centers for Disease Control and Prevention)
2. direct
3. OSHA (Occupational Safety and Health Administration)
4. hepatitis B virus (HBV)
5. titer
6. 5–10

Short Answer Questions

1. product name and identification by generic or trade name
   hazardous components
   potential health dangers
   potential for flammability or explosion
   spill or disposal procedures
   recommended or required PPE
   storage and handling guidelines
2. skin
   eyes
   mouth
   gastrointestinal tract
   respiratory tract
   genitourinary tract
3. moisture
   nutrients
   temperature
   darkness
   neutral to slightly alkaline pH environment
   oxygen
4. Hepatitis B is spread through health care professionals by contact with infected blood or body fluid.

Innovative Activities

Labeling
Refer to textbook Figure 1-1, Infection Cycle.

CHAPTER 2

Vocabulary

Definitions

1. signs
2. hereditary
3. familial
4. chief complaint
5. over-the-counter
6. symptoms
7. assessment

Matching

1. a
2. d
3. b
4. b
5. d
6. a or c (The smoking of cigarettes may be asked under past medical history, ROS or under social history, depending upon forms used or preference of physician.)
7. c

Skill Drills

1. identifying data or data base—patient's name and date of birth, address, home and work telephone number, insurance carrier and policy number, social security number, gender and race

   past history—allergies, immunizations, childhood diseases, current and past medications, previous illnesses, traumatic injuries, surgeries, and hospitalizations

   review of systems—thorough review of each body system to elicit information that the patient may have forgotten to mention or may have felt was irrelevant

   family history—health status of patient's family including specific diseases or disorders

   social history—information on patient's lifestyle, such as marital status, occupation, education and hobbies

2. S—subjective—information reported by the patient

   O—objective—information obtained from the health care worker's observation of the patient

   A—assessment—problem identification

   P—plan—proposed treatment

Innovative Activities

See Figure 2-1, Sample Medical History, with results written in a clear, concise, and objective manner.

Charting Exercise

Explain to Mrs. Adams that only authorized individuals can have access to patient information. If the information is to be transmitted to someone outside the medical office staff, the patient must sign a release of information form. Though the chart belongs to the facility, the information belongs to the patient to do with as he or she sees fit.

Complains of dizziness for the past 2 days, states fell and hit head 1 week ago and "wonders if the blow to the head could be causing dizziness now." Says takes no regular medication.

CHAPTER 3

Vocabulary

Word Scramble

1. cardinal signs
2. febrile
3. cardiac cycle
4. hypertension
5. remittent
6. diastole

Fill-in-the-Boxes

1. anthropometric
2. systole
3. intermittent
4. calibrated
5. postural hypotension
6. baseline

Charting Exercise

12/11/98 11:00 a.m.
62-yr-old male c/c routine physical examination BP 130/86 T-98.6 P 78 R 20

J. Adams, MA

Basic Writing Activities

Skill Drills

1. glass mercury thermometers—glass tube divided into two major parts, a glass column and the bulb filled with mercury and shaped in a long slender form for oral use and rounded stub form for rectal use. Heat expands the mercury, which rises in the glass column to measure degrees of temperature.

   electronic thermometers—portable battery-operated units with sheath-covered probes; temperature is sensed and a digital read-out is given in the window of the hand-held base.

   tympanic thermometers—battery-operated; fitted with a disposable cover and inserted in the ear much like an otoscope. A trigger is pulled or a button is pressed and an infrared light bounces off the tympanic membrane, recording the body's temperature on a digital screen in 2 seconds.

   disposable thermometers: single-use thermometers that register quickly with color changes on a strip placed against the skin.

2. Korotkoff sounds

   first sound—"lubb"—reflects the systolic period of cardiac cycle

   second sound—"dubb"—reflects the diastolic period of cardiac cycle

   "lubb-dubb"—one heart beat/one cardiac cycle of contraction and relaxation

Five phases of blood pressure/phase sounds

1. faint tapping sounds heard as the cuff deflates (systolic)
2. soft swishing sounds
3. rhythmic, sharp, distinct tapping sounds
4. soft tapping sounds that become faint
5. no sounds (diastolic)

3. Descriptions of respiratory rate

   bradypnea—slower than average

   tachypnea—much faster than the average

   dyspnea—difficult or labored breathing

   apnea—no respirations

   hyperpnea—abnormally deep, gasping breaths

   hyperventilation—a respiratory rate that greatly exceeds the oxygen demand

   hypopnea—shallow respirations

   orthopnea—inability to breathe or difficulty breathing in a supine or prone position; the patient usually has to sit upright to breathe

Innovative Activities

Labeling

See Figure 3-3, Four Glass Thermometers, in the text.
Centigrade oral—37.8° C
Centigrade rectal—40.0° C
Fahrenheit rectal—99.2° F
Fahrenheit oral—102.1° F

CHAPTER 4

Vocabulary

Definitions

1. the act of listening to sounds within the body
2. an abnormal sound or murmur heard in the blood vessels while auscultating an organ, gland, or blood vessel
3. a chemical substance used to bind, fix, or stabilize specimens of tissue to slides for later examination
4. visual examination
5. the act or process of measuring
6. hidden or concealed from observation
7. abbreviation used in documentation to denote pupils equal, round, reactive to light and accommodation if all findings are normal
8. the range, measured in degrees, through which a joint can be extended and flexed
9. the passage of light through body tissues for the purpose of examination

Matching

1. g 3. c 5. e 7. b
2. d 4. f 6. a

Case Studies

1. Explain to Mrs. Green that while the lithotomy position is the preferred position for a genital examination, the doctor can examine her in another position. The options are the dorsal recumbent position (supine with legs separated, knees bent and feet flat on the examination table) or the Sims' position (patient lies on left side with the left arm and shoulder behind the body, the right leg and arm sharply flexed on the table, and the left knee slightly flexed).
2. Steps to developing rapport with patients:

- Call patient by name from waiting room
- Escort patient to examination room
- Assess patient's facial expression and level of anxiety
- Note verbal and nonverbal behavior
- Speak clearly with a confident tone in voice
- Explain what is expected of the patient
- Explain procedures to patient
- Allow for questions
- Answer questions clearly and at a level that patient can understand

Charting Exercise

9/23/99 9:30 a.m.

65-yr-old female here for physical exam. Ht 5'7", Wt 135 lbs, BP 110/60, P 88

Urine specimen collected for urinalysis. 12 lead EKG done. Explained to patient UA and EKG part of routine prep for exam.

J. Adams, MA

Basic Writing Activities

Skill Drills

1. medical history
   actual physical examination
   laboratory and diagnostic tests
   perform follow-up treatments and procedures, if necessary
   direct the patient to dress
   return to examination room and ask patient if he or she has any questions
   reinforce any instructions that have been given and provide patient education
2. Instrument/Function—any four of the following:
   percussion hammer—test neurologic reflexes
   tuning fork—test hearing
   nasal speculum—visual inspection of the nose
   otoscope—visualization of the ear canal and tympanic membrane
   ophthalmoscope—examine the interior structures of the eye
   audio scope—screen patients for hearing loss
   examination light—increase illumination of area that physician is examining
   gooseneck lamp—provide illumination to specific area physician is examining
   tape measure—measure in inches and feet or centimeters and meters
   gloves—used when mouth, vagina, and rectum are examined to protect the patient and physician from microorganisms
   stethoscope—listening to body sounds
   tongue depressor—hold down the tongue to inspect the mouth and throat
   penlight and flashlight—provide light during the examination
   anoscope—instrument used to visualize the anal canal
   proctoscope—instrument used to visualize the rectum
   sigmoidoscope—instrument used to visualize the entire rectum, sigmoid colon, and possibly a portion of descending colon

Fill-in-the-Blanks

1. histobrush
2. any one of the following: palpation, rectal, vaginal, rectovaginal
3. lubricant
4. pearly gray
5. cerumen

Innovative Activities

Labeling

Refer to figures 4-1, 4-2, 4-3, 4-4, 4-5, 4-6, 4-7, 4-8, and 4-9 in text for the various medical instruments.

CHAPTER 5

Vocabulary

Matching

1. d 3. g 5. b 7. e
2. f 4. a 6. c

Definitions

1. an appliance used to sterilize medical instruments or other objects by steam under pressure
2. a chemical that can be applied to objects to destroy microorganisms; will not destroy bacterial spores
3. the process of killing or rendering inert most, but not all, pathogenic organisms
4. a chemical or drug that kills most pathogenic microorganisms
5. a mechanical implement
6. the practice of lowering the number of microorganisms on a surface by use of low-level disinfectant practices
7. a specific area, such as within a tray or on a sterile towel, that is considered free of microorganisms
8. a process, act, or technique for destroying microorganisms using heat, water, chemicals, or gases

Basic Writing Activities

Short Answer Questions

1. Disinfection destroys kills or renders inert most, but not all, pathogenic organisms while sterilization destroys all microorganisms including bacterial spores.
2. It is important to keep an up-to-date master list of all instruments and supplies, including all purchases and replacements, in order to maintain an adequate supply of instruments necessary for the practice and monitor costs of maintaining such a supply.

Skill Drills

1. hemostat clamp
   Kelly clamp
   sterilizer forceps
   needle holder
   spring or thumb forceps
2. be permeable to steam but not contaminants
   resist tearing and puncturing during normal handling
   allow easy opening to prevent contamination of the contents
   maintain sterility of the item during storage
3. date and time of the cycle
   general description of the contents of the load
   exposure time and temperature
   name or initials of the operator
   results of the sterilization indicator
   expiration date of the load (usually 30 days)
4. Any four of the following:
   alcohol (70% isopropyl alcohol or ethyl alcohol)
   chlorine (sodium hypochlorite or bleach)
   iodine or iodophores
   phenols
   formaldehyde
   hydrogen peroxide
   glutaraldehyde

Innovative Activities

Refer to Figure 5-2, Types of Scissors, in text.

CHAPTER 6

Vocabulary

Matching

1. c 3. a 5. b
2. d 4. e

Definitions

1. soft material applied to a body part for treatment purposes; usually a soft, absorbent gauze to hold a dressing, immobilize or support a part, aid in controlling bleeding
2. a covering applied directly to a wound to apply pressure or support, to absorb secretions, to protect from trauma or microorganisms, to stop or slow bleeding or to hide disfigurement
3. a substance that delays decomposition
4. notched mechanisms, usually at the handle end of an instrument, that click into position to maintain tension on the opposing blades or tips of the instrument
5. a medium for conducting or detecting electrical current
6. a metal needle fused to suture material

Case Studies

1. Apply to the wound the number of sterile dressings needed to properly cover and protect the wound (sterile 2x2s or 4x4s are possible choices); apply the bandage so that it completely covers the sterile dressing and conforms to the patient's contours (i.e., sterile gauze roll). There are a number of different dressing and bandage types, therefore the MA should ask the physician for his/her preference or choice. Sterile techniques should be utilized throughout the procedure.

2. Explain to Mr. Johnson that the simplest form of healing results from wounds that are closely approximated (as his has been with sutures). allowing the entrance of little or no bacteria to complicate the process. The edges of the wound lie closely together, new cells form quickly to bind the site, and capillaries expand themselves across the tissue break to restore circulation to the tissues. There is usually little scarring. (The process you have explained is known as healing by primary intention.) Explain the phases of wound healing: phase 1 (inflammatory phase), where the body tries to heal itself by increasing circulation and white blood cells to the injured area and the wound edges comes closer together and form a scab (approximate time in this phase is 1–4 days); phase 2 (healing phase), where the vessels continue to heal themselves and the scab continues to dry and pull wound edges closely together; phase 3 (remodeling phase), which may take from weeks to years, depending on the severity of the wound, and in which scar tissue is formed to guard the site.

Give Mr. Johnson the following instructions in order for him to protect the wound during dressing changes at home, and further explain to him that these steps are necessary to avoid compromising the healing process and spreading pathogens.

1. Wash hands before and after each dressing change.
2. Use gloves for dressing changes, and use clean or aseptic technique as well as impervious bags to hold old dressings.
3. Apply dressings and bandage as demonstrated in the office, or as directed by the physician.
4. Dressing and bandages are to be kept clean and dry.
5. Report increased drainage, odor, redness, swelling, increased pain, or fever.
6. Return as directed for office rechecks or for suture removal.

Charting Exercise

11/12/00 10:00 a.m.
Educated to wound healing and instructed in dressing changes.
Advised to report signs of infection and given date for suture removal.

John White, RMA

Basic Writing Activities

Fill-in-the-Blanks

1. transversely
2. medically aseptic
3. repackaged and resterilized
4. void
5. fulguration
6. sterile

Skill Drills

1. Do not let sterile packages become damp or wet.
   Always face a sterile field.
   Hold all sterile items above waist level.
   Place sterile items in the middle of the sterile field.
   Do not spill any liquids, even sterile liquids, onto the sterile field.
   Do not cough, sneeze, or talk over the sterile field.
   Never reach over the sterile field.
   Be aware that soiled supplies, such as gauze or instruments, should not be passed over or placed on the sterile field.
   If you know or suspect that the sterile field has been contaminated, alert the physician.
2. Any three of the following:
   lidocaine (Xylocaine, Baylocaine)
   Xylocaine with epinephrine
   mepivacaine (Carbocaine)
   bupivacaine (Marcaine)
3. using sterile transfer forceps
   using the sterile gloved hand
   flipping the contents onto a sterile field
4. applying pressure to control bleeding
   holding a dressing in place
   protecting dressings and wounds from contamination
   immobilizing an injured part of the body
   supporting an injured part of the body

Innovative Activities

Labeling

Refer to Box 6-2 in text.

Primary Intention: clean incision, early suture, hairline scar

Secondary Intention: gaping irregular wound, granulation, epithelium grows over scar

Tertiary Intention: wound, increased granulation, late suturing with wide scar

CHAPTER 7

Vocabulary

Matching

1. h	3. i	5. f	7. d	9. c
2. g	4. a	6. b	8. e	

Word Scramble

1. drug
2. potentiation
3. synergism
4. pharmacology
5. antagonism
6. pharmacodynamics
7. pharmacokinesis

Case Studies

Diazepam (Valium) is a Schedule IV medication. Schedule IV drugs may be filled up to five times in a 6-month period. Mrs. Smith's original Rx was written on 4/19/99 and refilled four times as of 11/19/99. She has had a total of five prescriptions in seven months. This time frame falls within the limits for Schedule IV drugs. Mrs. Smith would be able to receive a refill if the physician is willing to write one.

Tylenol with codeine is a Schedule III medication. As such it is considered to have a limited potential for psychological or physiological dependence. The medical assistant should tell the patient that while the drug has some potential for addiction, the physician feels that it is appropriate to use it at this time for pain management. The medical assistant should instruct Mr. Jones to take it only as directed and if necessary for pain management. The medical assistant should also instruct Mr. Jones to contact the physician if his pain is not relieved by the medication.

Charting Exercise

12/1/99 1:00 p.m.
Refill approved by MD for Benadryl 50mg #30 1 tab po qid PRN
Allergies (called into pharmacy)

J. Adams, MA

Basic Writing Activities

Skill Drills

1. redness and swelling at the injection site
   itching, either at the site or generalized
   dyspnea
   nausea
   dizziness
2. Physician's Desk Reference (PDR)
   United States Pharmacopeia Dispensing Information (USPDI)
   American Hospital Formulary Service (AHFS)
   Compendium of Drug Therapy
3. Pure Food and Drug Act (1906)
   Federal Food, Drug, and Cosmetic Act (1938)
   Durham-Humphrey Amendment (1952)
   Kefauver-Harris Amendment (1962)
4. age
   weight
   sex
   existing pathology
   tolerance

Fill-in-the-Blanks

1. 17
2. 1906, 1938
3. chemical
4. generic
5. actions, effects

Innovative Activities

Labeling

Refer to Figure 7-1, Sample Prescription Form.
Show this sample prescription and identify the seven parts (omit generic option) by number and leave a blank next to number for student to identify part, i.e., date, inscription.

CHAPTER 8

Vocabulary

Matching

1. g 3. a 5. i 7. e 9. c
2. h 4. f 6. b 8. d 10. j

Definitions

1. a small glass container that can be sealed and its contents sterilized
2. an agent that dilutes the substance or solution to which it is added
3. a standard of measurement; a device for measuring size, capacity amount, or power of an object or substance
4. tuberculin skin test using a purified protein derivative (PPD) of tuberculin bacillus given intradermally to establish exposure to tuberculosis
5. the curved upper surface of a liquid in a container
6. an instrument for administering a fine spray of medication, usually used in the respiratory tract
7. a small bottle for medicine or chemicals

Case Studies

1. Explain to Mr. Alexander that a tine test is used for routine screening and tests for the presence of tuberculin antibodies. A positive tine test is usually followed by a Mantoux test (which is more diagnostic). A positive Mantoux reaction will indicate the possibility of active or dormant tuberculosis or exposure to the disease. Mr. Alexander needs to be instructed to return to the office in 48 to 72 hours for an evaluation of the test site.

2. You will give 1/2 tablet. Ratio-proportion should be set up:
400mg:1 tablet :: 200mg:X tablet
400× divided into 200 = .5
X = .5 tablets

Charting Exercise

5/6/00 10:00 a.m.
Tagamet 200mg given PO per Dr. Matthew's order.

Sharon Kline, CMA

Basic Writing Activities

Skill Drills

1. intradermal injections: 10–15-degree angle
subcutaneous injections: 45-degree angle
intramuscular injections: 90-degree angle
2. mark through the charting error with one line
mark the correction above the error
sign your name next to the correction
3. right patient
right time and frequency of administration
right dose
right route of administration
right drug
right technique
right documentation
4. date of the reconstitution
initials of the person who reconstituted the drug
diluent used

Completion

1. 1 ml
2. 2.2
3. 1 inch
4. 25g ⅝ inch or 23g ½ inch
5. ampules
6. 15 or 16

Innovative Activities

Labeling

Parts of a syringe and needle (see Figure 8-8):
plunger
barrel
needle hilt
needle
bevel
shaft lumen

CHAPTER 9

Vocabulary

Matching

1. e 3. c 5. b 7. f
2. g 4. d 6. a

Definitions

1. standing position with the body erect, facing forward, feet pointed forward and slightly apart, arms down at the sides with the palms facing forward and the thumbs outward
2. the study of the body's structure
3. a substance made up of only one type of atom
4. the study of the body's functions
5. an imaginary line drawn through the body and used to facilitate the study of individual organs or the body as a whole
6. four parts; used as a way to divide the abdomen into four parts
7. groups of organs that work together to perform a specific function for the body

Case Studies

1. The terms used by the medical assistant are medical terms used to describe the size and location of the cut on Jack's arm.
2. Right hypochondriac region: Because the abdominal cavity is so large an area, it is divided into nine areas, called abdominal regions, to provide a more accurate means of identifying underlying organ and structure locations.

Charting Exercise

10/25/99 2:30 p.m.
45-yr-old female with c/o rt hypochondriac pain x 1 wk, especially pc, some nausea, no diarrhea.

S. Crane, MA

Basic Writing Activities

Skill Drills

1. cranial cavity
   spinal cavity
   thoracic cavity
   abdominal cavity
   pelvic cavity
2. heart
   lungs
   esophagus
   trachea
3. Standing with the body erect, facing forward, feet pointed forward and slightly apart, arms down at the sides with the palms facing forward and the thumbs outward
4. right hypochondriac region
   epigastric region
   left hypochondriac region
   right lumbar region
   umbilical region
   left lumbar region
   right iliac region
   hypogastric region
   left iliac region

Fill-in-the-Blanks

1. cell
2. organs
3. nine
4. positive feedback
5. cell membrane, cytoplasm, nucleus
6. atom, element

Innovative Activities

Refer to Figure 9-7, Cavities of the Body.

CHAPTER 10

Vocabulary

Matching

1. e 3. b 5. a
2. d 4. c

Definitions

1. an inflamed cavity filled with pus as a result of infection
2. blackheads associated with acne vulgaris
3. cracks in the skin
4. raised, solid lesion larger than 1 cm
5. hives
6. a fungal infection of the skin

Case Studies

1. You will prepare Miss Smith for the examination by:
   a. exposing and draping the patient's left anterior thigh
   b. assembling a sterile culture tube (with swab), a lab requisition slip, and any other equipment and supplies the doctor may have requested
   c. appropriately positioning the lighting
2. Educate Mr. and Mrs. Connors to the purpose, performance, and expected outcomes of applying (warm) compresses.

   Purpose
   - Hasten healing by increasing blood flow to a part.
   - Relieve pain.
   - Relieve muscle spasm or tension.
   - Provide for local warming.

   Performance
   - Temperature should be from tepid 95/98 degrees, to a very warm 115 degrees.
   - Wear gloves (sterile gloves if the condition requires).
   - Place a pad under the body part to catch drips.
   - Check for patient response to temperature when the compress is first applied.
   - Insulate the compress with a waterproof barrier (this will retard heat loss).
   - Heat should be applied for no longer than 30 minutes and not repeated for at least 1 hour afterward.
   - Apply compresses according to the physician's direction (in this case it is three times per day).

   Expected Outcomes
   - Healing will be hastened.
   - Pain will be relieved.
   - Muscle spasm or tension will be relieved.
   - Procedure will be tolerated with no adverse effects.

   Precautions
   - Do not increase water temperature when the patient has adapted to the temperature—a burn may occur.
   - Do not leave the warm compress on longer than 30 minutes—after 30 minutes there is an opposite effect.
   - The very young and the elderly are more prone to burn, therefore it is important to frequently check the body part, and the compress temperature.
   - Report any excess redness, pain, or swelling.

Charting Exercise

10/10/00 10:30 a.m.

Left anterior thigh draped for examination. Culture specimen collected from drainage of wound on the left anterior thigh, and sent to the lab.

Kelly Jones, CMA

Basic Writing Activities

Skill Drills

1. epidermis
   dermis
   subcutaneous tissue
2. protection—unbroken skin provides a protective barrier that prevents the entrance of microorganisms and is the body's first line of defense against infection. It also protects the body from mechanical injury, damaging substances, and the ultraviolet rays of the sun.

   regulation of body temperature—increased sweat production in a warm environment lowers body temperature as sweat evaporates. Blood vessels in the skin dilate, bringing interior heat close to the body's surface to cool the body. In a cold environment, the blood vessels constrict to conserve heat.

   sensation—receptors for heat, cold, pain, touch, and pressure
3. Any four of the following:
   - foods such as shellfish, strawberries, tomatoes, citrus fruit, eggs, and chocolate
   - inhalants such as feathers or animal dander
   - chemicals, cosmetics, and medications
   - sunlight
   - insect bites or stings
   - heat, cold, or pressure on the skin
   - infection
   - stress
4. injectable epinephrine with syringes and needles
   various sizes of airways and intubation devices
   oxygen and masks or ambu bags
   tourniquet

Fill-in-the-Blanks

1. basal cell carcinoma
2. 15
3. sweat
4. D
5. staphylococcus or streptococcus

Innovative Activities

Students should visit a physician's office and obtain examples of educational brochures, or perhaps the instructors will have examples to look at for reference. A medical educational brochure should be clear, concise, and written in common language so that patients can understand.

CHAPTER 11

Vocabulary

Matching

1. d 3. f 5. c 7. e
2. g 4. a 6. b

Definitions

1. amphiarthrosis
2. antagonist
3. arthroplasty
4. contracture
5. synergist
6. goniometer
7. electromyography

Case Studies

1. Fractures heal by callus formation at the site of the fracture. The callus holds the ends of the bones together; with time the callus turns to bone. Bone cells mold the callus and smooth the fracture site to close to its original size. Immobilization of the fracture by casting and support with a sling allows the molding and reshaping process to take place successfully.
2. *Tendonitis*

Definition: an inflammation of tendons

Cause: occurs after strains, sprains, overuse, or overstretching of the tissue

Symptoms: local tenderness; pain occurs with active movement and resistance to movement is intensely painful because the tissue must contract during active and resisted movement

Treatment: rest, heat or cold applications, ultrasound, iontophoresis, massage, and deep massage across the fibers of the tendons; medications as ordered by your physician

Charting Exercise

10/28/99 10:00 a.m.
9-yr-old boy with fracture of lt arm. Fracture reduced and cast applied.
10/28/99 10:20 a.m.
Fingers left hand warm to touch and pink in color. Triangle sling applied.
Instructions to mother to check circulation to left hand frequently and use sling for support.

Alice Worth, MA

Basic Writing Activities

Skill Drills

1. long bones—largest bones in the body, making up most of the appendicular skeleton

   short bones—generally more equal in height, length, and width; usually articulate with more than one bone

   flat bones—thin bones with broad surfaces; are more curved than flat

   sesamoid bones—small bones that develop within tendons

   irregular bones—mixed shapes and varieties that do not fit into the other categories
2. kyphosis—abnormal thoracic curvature, particularly the upper portion (hunchback)

   lordosis—abnormal deep lumbar curvature (swayback)

   scoliosis—side-to-side or lateral curve
3. hyaline cartilage—articular cartilage, covering ends of opposing bones; has no blood supply and gets its nutrients from the synovial fluid; cannot heal itself when damaged

   fibro cartilage—a shock absorber, fills the gap between two bones

   elastic cartilage—allows for specific movements
4. Any four of the following:

   simple or closed—a break in the bone that does not protrude through the skin

   compound or open—a break in the bone in which the broken end protrudes through the skin

   spiral—a fracture that occurs with torsion or twisting-type injuries

   impacted—a fracture in which one bone segment is driven into another

   greenstick—a common injury in children involving a partial or incomplete break in which only one side of a bone is broken like a green stick

   transverse—a fracture that is at right angles to the axis of the bone

   oblique—a fracture that is slanted across the axis of the bone

   comminuted—a fracture occurring when a bone is fragmented

   compression—results from damage to the bone by the application of strong force against both ends

   depressed—a fracture of flat bones causing the fragment to be driven below the surface of the bone

   avulsion—a fracture caused by a strong force applied to the bone by the sharp, twisting/pulling motion of the attached ligaments or tendons

   pathologic—fractures that are usually a result of disease processes such as osteoporosis (brittle bones)

Short Answer Questions

1. chondromalacia patellae
2. bunions, corns, calluses
3. Osteoarthritis is caused by wear and tear on the weight-bearing joints in which the articular cartilage degenerates and the ends of the bones enlarge. Rheumatoid arthritis is a systemic autoimmune disease that attacks the synovium of the joint, ultimately leading to inflammation, pain, stiffness, and crippling deformities.
4. bottom of the foot
5. wrist
6. fingers

Innovative Activities

Refer to Figure 11-3, Normal Range of Motion of Selected Joints.

CHAPTER 12

Vocabulary

Matching

1. b 3. e 5. c 7. f
2. d 4. a 6. g

Word Scramble

1. pons
2. sulci
3. cranium
4. autonomic
5. arachnoid

Case Studies

1. You can tell Mr. Mendoza that migraine headaches are one of the most common types of headaches. They can be triggered by stress, high altitude, smoking, certain smells, or ingested chemicals (caffeine, alcohol, certain food additives), but in many situations the cause is unknown. Patients who have migraines may complain of an aura before the onset. Symptoms usually include a unilateral temporal headache, photophobia, diplopia, and nausea. Generally headaches are treated with analgesics, and the patient may be instructed to rest in a dark, quiet room.

2. Explain to Ms. Winters that seizures are treated with various pharmacologic agents and have her direct her questions on this matter to the doctor. You may tell Ms. Winters that a patient who has seizures is allowed to have a driver's license; however, each state has specific regulations requiring that patients be seizure free for a particular length of time (e.g., 2 years) to qualify.

Charting Exercise

2/25/00 3:30 p.m.

CC: sudden onset of a "terrible headache on the left side of the head," "nausea," and states that bright lights in the exam room hurt his eyes. T. 99 degrees P. 88 R. 24 BP 138/86.

Diane Williams, CMA

2/25/00 3:50 p.m.

Medicated per physician order. (Note: this would be filled in with the name of the medication, dose, and route given.) Resting quietly in a darkened room, waiting for wife to arrive to take home.

Diane Williams, CMA

2/25/00 4:40 p.m.

Information given regarding migraines. Leaves with wife, she to drive home.

Diane Williams, CMA

Basic Writing Activities

Skill Drills

1. cerebrum—largest part of the brain, divided into two hemispheres, responsible for thought process, sensory and motor function, speech, writing, memory, and emotions.

   brain stem—composed of midbrain, pons, medulla oblongata; the midbrain serves primarily as a relay center for messages that control certain eye and ear reflexes; the pons is responsible for communication within the central nervous system; the medulla oblongata controls breathing, heart rate, and blood pressure.

   cerebellum—responsible for balance and muscle coordination
2. hemiplegia—paralysis on one side of the body opposite involvement

   paraplegia—paralysis of any part of the body below the point of involvement

   quadriplegia—paralysis of all limbs
3. meningitis

   encephalitis

   poliomyelitis

   tetanus

   rabies

   Reye's syndrome
4. Multiple sclerosis (MS)

   Physical: The myelin sheaths degenerate and are replaced with plaques which impair nerve impulse conduction. Typically patients will present with complaints of progressive loss of muscle control. They may also complain of loss of balance, shaking tremors, and poor muscle coordination. Tingling and numbness can also be first signs. Dysphagia may be another symptom. As the disease progresses, bladder dysfunction and visual complaints are common. Patients may also develop nystagmus.

   Emotional: This disease affects persons in the "prime of life." Patients must struggle with emotional concerns regarding long-term welfare of the family.

   Amyotrophic lateral sclerosis (Lou Gehrig's disease)

   Physical: Causes progressive loss of motor neurons. It is a terminal disease with no known etiology; there is a strong familial connection. Typically is seen most often in middle-aged men. It begins with loss of muscle mobility in the forearms, hands, and legs, then progresses to the face muscles, causing dysphagia and dysphasia that worsen over time. Death usually occurs in 3 to 5 years after the onset of symptoms.

   Emotional: This disease affects person in the "prime of life." Patients must struggle with emotional concerns regarding long-term welfare of family and death within 3 to 5 years.

Fill-in-the-Blanks

1. efferent
2. afferent
3. neurotransmitter
4. parasympathetic system
5. lock jaw

Innovative Activities

Labeling

Refer to Figure 12-2, Diagram of Motor Neuron, in text.

CHAPTER 13

Vocabulary

Matching

1. d 3. f 5. b 7. c
2. e 4. g 6. a

Definitions

1. an accessory structure or part
2. ear wax
3. a unit for measuring the intensity of sound
4. a trained specialist who grinds lenses to fit refraction
5. a trained specialist who can measure for errors of refraction and prescribe lenses
6. bending of light as it enters the eye
7. pertaining to the sense of touch

Case Studies

"Swimmers ear" or otitis externa is an inflammation or infection of the external ear. It is common among swimmers whose ear canals are exposed to moisture. The warm, moist ear canal is a perfect environment for pathogens. Advising the use of ear plugs will prevent exposure to moisture.

A Snellen chart is generally used to test visual acuity. When checking the vision of a 5-year-old the medical assistant will need to ascertain the child's capacity to read or recognize letters. If the child does not know the alphabet, then the "E" or object chart may be used. The medical assistant should take time to familiarize the child with the chart. Also, the medical assistant should test the child at 10 feet rather than 20 feet as children have difficulty focusing and at 10 feet there is less opportunity for distraction in the line of vision.

Charting Exercise

9/4/99 10:00 a.m.
17-yr-old with left ear pain x 2 days and jaw pain. Dx: Otitis Externa, left ear. Rx: Amoxicillin 250mg. Aid x 10 days.

M. Berg, MA

Basic Writing Activities

Skill Drills

1. scleral-corneal layer—sclera forms the outer cover of the eye and is connected to the cornea, the anterior one-sixth of the eye. The cornea is transparent and covers the iris and pupil. It refracts light as it enters the eye.
   choroid layer—vascular layer of the interior of the eye that absorbs light when it enters the eye
   retina—innermost portion of the eye that functions primarily to form images
   intrinsic (inside) muscles—change the shape of the lens for refraction and the pupil for the entrance of light
   extrinsic (outside) muscles—responsible for eye movement and must coordinate movements in the field of vision
2. Snellen chart
   Jeager chart
3. heredity with predisposing factors to deafness
   infections
   trauma
   ototoxic drugs
   neurologic diseases
   exposure to loud noises

Fill-in-the-Blanks

1. hordeolum
2. bacteria
3. fungi
4. viruses
5. protozoa
6. trauma
7. allergens
8. toxins
9. pinna, auricle, external
10. hearing, equilibrium
11. stapes

Innovative Activities

Labeling

Refer to Figure 13-16, Organs of Taste and Smell.

CHAPTER 14

Vocabulary

Matching

1. e 3. c 5. a
2. d 4. b

Definitions

1. a disease that occurs continuously in a particular population but has a low mortality; used in contrast to epidemic
2. an enlargement of the thyroid gland
3. the presence of glucose in the urine
4. excessive proliferation of normal cells in the normal tissue arrangement of an organism
5. the most severe form of hypothyroidism; signs include edema of the extremities and the face
6. excessive thirst
7. itching
8. severe cramping, convulsions, or muscle spasm due to an abnormality of calcium metabolism

Case Studies

1. Explain to Mrs. Walker the difference between type I and type II diabetes mellitus:

   Type I—occurs most often in children and young adults. Onset of type I is abrupt, with symptoms such as polyuria, polydipsia, polyphagia (abnormal hunger), weight loss, and ketoacidosis (acidosis accompanied by an accumulation ketones [end product of fat metabolism] in the body). Insulin must be administered parenterally to control type I diabetes.

   Type II—occurs most often in adults over age 40. Onset of type II is gradual, with symptoms such as polyuria, polydipsia, pruritus (severe itching), and peripheral neuropathy. In this condition, insulin is produced but cannot exert its effect on cells because of a deficiency of insulin receptors on cell membranes. Risk factors are obesity and family history of diabetes. Control of type II diabetes may not require insulin. The patient is usually placed on a well-balanced diet, adequate in all basic essentials; carbohydrates, proteins, fats, vitamins, minerals, and fluids. Obese patients must be placed on a diet that will enable them to lose weight. Controlling diabetes is difficult in an obese person. When the patient is given an adequate diet and glucose still appears in the urine, insulin may be required. Oral drugs that enable insulin to react with the remaining cell membrane receptors have been used successfully in middle-aged and older patients.
2. Educate Mr. Allison to the importance of the relationship between insulin injections and eating. You tell Mr. Allison that the relationship between eating and insulin injections is very important. Include in your explanation:

   Insulin shock—occurs from an overdose or overproduction of insulin. This results in blood sugar levels well below normal. Skipping a meal without adjusting insulin levels will also result in insulin shock. Review insulin shock signs and symptoms with Mr. Allison.

   Diabetic coma—results from lack of insulin. This condition causes metabolic changes with excess production of ketone bodies. Review diabetic ketoacidosis with Mr. Allison.

   Give Mr. Allison written materials regarding diabetes mellitus. You may also tell him that the American Diabetes Association has a broad selection of printed materials to help diabetic patients adjust to lifestyle changes. Type I diabetic individuals may need a support group to learn to incorporate medical compliance into their lives with as little disruption as possible.

Charting Exercise

3/10/00 2:00 p.m.
Has successfully learned how to self-administer insulin. Questions timing of injections and meals. Explained that the relationship between eating and insulin injections is very important and reviewed the signs and symptoms of insulin shock and diabetic coma. Written materials on diabetes mellitus given. Directed to the American Diabetes Association for additional written materials and support group information if wanted.

Doris Fry, RMA

Skill Drills

1. Diabetic coma results from lack of insulin. Insulin shock occurs from an overdose or overproduction of insulin.
2. Diabetes insipidus—results from hyposecretion of antidiuretic hormone (ADH) in the posterior pituitary. Deficient ADH causes the renal tubules to reabsorb little of the water and salts resulting in as much as 5–10 liters of urine output a day (polyuria). Clinical symptoms also include polydipsia as the body's effort to restore fluid balance. The cause is not usually known but may be due to head trauma or tumor formation. Treatment involves correction of the causative factor and the administration of synthetic ADH by injection or by nasal spray for vascular absorption.
3. Estrogen is produced by the follicle cells in the ovaries. Estrogen stimulates:

   maturation of the ova

   proliferation of blood vessels in the endometrium

   development of secondary sexual characteristics

   growth of the duct system of the mammary glands

   growth of the uterus

   disposition of fat subcutaneously in the hips and thighs
4. Ketoacidosis is a serious problem for patients with IDDM. When glucose cannot be used for energy, the body turns to fats and proteins, which the liver converts to ketones. Ketones accumulate in the blood because the cells cannot use them rapidly; as these organic acids build up, they lower the pH of the blood. The kidneys will excrete excess ketones, but in doing so will excrete more water. This excess excretion of water will lead to dehydration, worsening the acidosis.

   The administration of insulin is necessary to permit the use of glucose for energy. Intravenous fluids are used to restore blood volume to normal. If left untreated, ketoacidosis will progress to coma and death.

Completion

1. ductless
2. hypophysis or master gland
3. calcitonin
4. brain
5. testes and ovaries

Innovative Activities

New employee information sheets, regarding any subject, will vary from one facility to another. The student should visit a medical office and obtain an example (or obtain one from the instructor), then using the textbook develop their own information sheet regarding the various laboratory tests and diagnostic procedures that may be used to identify endocrine disorders.

CHAPTER 15

Vocabulary

Matching

1. b 3. f 5. g 7. c
2. d 4. a 6. e

Definitions

1. a localized dilation on a vessel wall
2. activity recorded on an electrocardiogram caused by patient movement, loose leads, or electrical interference
3. progressive wave of stimulation causing contraction of the myocardium
4. the condition of having the heart in the right side of the thoracic cavity
5. electrodes or electrical connections attached to the body to record electrical impulses in the body, especially the heart or brain
6. the mid-portion of the thoracic cavity containing the heart, the great vessels, the upper esophagus, and the trachea
7. the active process of restoring the cardiac fibers to the resting (polarized) state; reestablishment of the electrical polarized state in a muscle or nerve fiber following contraction or conduction of a nerve impulse

Case Studies

1. In many instances cardiac problems may not be apparent during a brief ECG. For diagnosis of intermittent cardiac arrhythmias and dysfunctions, a Holter monitor is worn for 24 hours. The monitor can be programmed to record for the full 24 hours or it may be programmed to record when the patient presses a record button at the onset of symptoms.
2. A cardiac stress test is performed with the patient attached to an ECG monitor. The patient is exposed to increased demand on the myocardium by walking on a treadmill or riding a stationary bicycle. The ECG provides a constant tracing from which the physician may diagnose any abnormalities. A thallium scan may also be performed in conjunction with the stress test. An isotope, thallium, is injected intravenously and localizes in the myocardium. A scintigraphy machine produces two-dimensional images that reveal any occlusions of the coronary arteries. Both tests are performed only when a physician is present and emergency equipment is available. Patients can be assured that the physician will be present and if they have discomfort the test will be stopped.

Charting Exercise

8/30/99 3:30 p.m.
After explanation of tests, cardiac stress test and thallium scan performed with physician present.

B. Maul, RMA

Basic Writing Activities

Skill Drills

1. An electrical impulse travels through the heart in the following way:
   SA node
   AV node
   bundle of His
   Purkinje fibers
2. mild numbness in the face or limb
   difficulty swallowing
   coughing and choking
   slurred speech
   unilateral visual disturbances
   dizziness
3. carditis—any of the layers of the heart muscle
   pericarditis—sac surrounding the heart muscle
   myocarditis—diffused throughout heart muscle or localized
   endocarditis—lining of the heart and its valves
4. trauma
   hypertension
   atherosclerosis
   fungal infections
   syphilis
   congenital defects

Fill-in-the-Blanks

1. coronary artery disease
2. 140/90
3. aortic stenosis
4. varicose veins
5. Doppler ultrasonography

Innovative Activities

Labeling

Refer to Figure 15-1, Heart and Great Vessels.

CHAPTER 16

Vocabulary

Matching

1. b 3. d 5. c 7. a
2. f 4. e 6. g

Word Scramble

1. vaccine
2. titer
3. macrophage
4. phagocyte
5. toxoid

Case Studies

1. Explain to Mr. Jones that patients who are HIV positive are treated prophylactically based on laboratory data. One parameter that is continuously monitored is the CD4 count. The CD4 is a surface molecule on the T cell. When HIV enters the body, it attaches to these molecules and destroys them, causing the CD4 count to fall. Treatment begins as the CD4 count falls, whether or not the patient has symptoms. As the CD4 count falls, further prophylactic antibiotic therapy may be started.

2. Give Miss Adams the name of the tests, and explain that the ELISA, or enzyme-linked immunosorbent assay, is used to screen blood for antibodies to the AIDS virus. A positive result indicates probable exposure to the virus and the possibility that the virus is in the blood. Since false-positive results can occur with the ELISA test, the Western blot test is used to confirm positive findings and is considered to be diagnostic.

Educate Miss Adams about the transmission of HIV by telling her to:

Avoid contact with another person's blood, body fluids, semen, or vaginal secretions.

Avoid sharing needles or syringes, or any objects that come in contact with blood or body fluids.

Avoid using alcohol or drugs. Use of these substances can hinder clear thinking and lead to unwise decision making.

You may also give her written patient education brochures or office materials regarding the transmission of HIV.

Charting Exercise

5/10/00 11:20 a.m.
Asks about CD4 testing and how it relates to treatment. Educated to general information regarding CD4 testing and explained that the physician uses the results to determine when treatment will start as well as how treatment may be managed. Blood for CD4 test drawn and sent to lab.

Jay Morgan, CMA

Basic Writing Activities

Skill Drills

1. List a minimum of two from each of the following groups:
   Lymphatic disorders
   - lymphangitis
   - elephantiasis
   - lymphadenitis
   - mononucleosis
   - splenomegaly
   - Hodgkin's disease
   - lymphosarcoma

   Immune system disorders
   - allergies
   - infantile hypogammaglobulinemia
   - acquired immunodeficiency syndrome
2. HIV—human immunodeficiency virus
   AIDS—acquired immunodeficiency syndrome
3. acute infectious stage, with generally mild, flu-like symptoms
   latent period, without symptoms
   complains of weight loss
   lymphadenopathy, fever, diarrhea, anorexia, fatigue, and skin rashes
   onset of immunodeficiency disorders such as Kaposi's sarcoma, and pneumocystis carinii pneumonia (possibly the initial stages of full-blown AIDS)
4. Exchange of body fluids that may result from sexual contact, sharing contaminated needles, transfusions of contaminated blood or accidental injury from sharp instruments used in invasive procedures; it also may be spread transplacentally from an infected mother to her infant.

Fill-in-the-Blanks

1. lymph
2. lymph nodes and nodules
3. tonsils
4. spleen
5. lymphangitis

Innovative Activities

Labeling

Refer to Figure 16-1, The Lymphatic System, for labeling answers listed on diagram.

CHAPTER 17

Vocabulary

Matching

1. c 3. g 5. b 7. d
2. f 4. a 6. e

Word Scramble

1. dyspnea
2. cilia
3. tonsils
4. carina
5. pleura
6. epiglottis

Case Studies

1. A peak flowmeter is an instrument used every day by the patient who has asthma. The peak flowmeter helps the patient assess their breathing and to determine what medication regimen to use that day. The physician designs a medication regimen that corresponds to the status of the patient's breathing as recorded with the peak flowmeter.
2. The purpose of a throat culture is to identify pathogens present in the throat that are causing tine inflammation or infection. The identity of these pathogens enables the physician to institute treatment if necessary.

Charting Exercise

9/6/99 1:30 p.m.
Patient c/o fever to 102 (orally) x 2 days, cough x 1 day, and sore throat x 3 days. Throat culture ordered by Dr. Jones.
9/8/99 9:30 a.m.
Throat culture obtained and sent to lab.

N. Lawson, MA

Basic Writing Activities

Skill Drills

1. External respiration is the exchange of gases between the alveoli and the pulmonary capillaries within the lungs. Internal respiration is the exchange of gases between the systemic capillaries, located throughout the body, and the cells of the body.
2. facilitate long-term ventilation
   relieve upper airway obstruction
   provide an airway after a laryngectomy
   facilitate suctioning in a patient who is unable to cough effectively
   decrease "dead space ventilation" in patients with chronic obstructive pulmonary disease
3. pharyngeal tonsils—nasopharyngeal space on the back wall of the upper pharynx
   palatine tonsils—back of the oral cavity
   lingual tonsils—at the base of the tongue

Fill-in-the-Blanks

1. morning
2. middle ear
3. 300
4. common cold, viruses or hay fever, allergens
5. lung fields
6. epiglottis, trachea

Innovative Activities

Labeling

Refer to Figure 17-2, Location of Paranasal Sinuses.

CHAPTER 18

Vocabulary

Matching

1. g 3. a 5. b 7. f
2. d 4. e 6. c

Definitions

1. the accumulation of serous fluid in the peritoneal cavity
2. a mobile mass
3. milky, fatty product of digestion absorbed through the small intestines and returned to circulation by the lymphatics
4. substance used to test for occult blood in the stool
5. black, tarry stools caused by digested blood from the GI tract
6. extreme constipation

Case Studies

1. Bowel preparation brochure will include the following:

Liquid diet without dairy products for the full day before the procedure or a clear liquid evening meal.

A laxative the evening preceding the procedure; enemas also may be ordered.

NPO except water after midnight through the time of the procedure.

Rectal suppository, Fleet's enema, or cleansing enema the morning of the procedure.

2. Explain to Mr. Zamora that a bowel study, such as a barium enema, requires that the bowel be completely clear of fecal matter for the test to be diagnostic, and that it is very important to carefully follow the bowel preparation directions.

Charting Exercise

12/14/00 2:30 p.m.
Scheduled for a barium enema on 12/17/00. T. 98.6 P. 80 R. 16 BP 120/80. Bowel preparation brochure given, and reviewed.

Barbara Martin, RMA

12/14/00 5:15 p.m.
Called in and questions if a light regular meal would be fine the day before the scheduled barium enema. Explained that the bowel must be free of fecal matter for the test to be diagnostic and that the bowel preparation directions must be carefully followed.

Barbara Martin, RMA

Basic Writing Activities

Skill Drills

1. cardiac region—the upper curve of the stomach near the heart
   fundus—balloons above the cardiac region
   body—middle or main portion
   antrum or pyloris—narrows to the pyloric sphincter
2. mouth
   oral pharynx
   esophagus
   stomach
   small intestines
   large intestine
3. liver
   gallbladder
   pancreas
4. Crohn's disease
   ulcerative colitis
   irritable bowel syndrome
   diverticulosis
   polyps
   hemorrhoids
   colorectal cancers

Completion Exercises

1. metabolism
2. stomatitis
3. gingivitis
4. ulcerative colitis
5. hemorrhoids

Innovative Activities

Labeling

Refer to Figures 18-1 and 18-2, The Gastrointestinal System and The Abdominal Cavity.

CHAPTER 19

Vocabulary

Matching

1. e 3. f 5. i 7. a 9. d
2. c 4. g 6. h 8. b

Definitions

1. a substance occurring in the blood that works with renin to affect the blood pressure, usually increasing the pressure by vasoconstriction
2. a hormone produced mainly by the kidney in response to lowered oxygen levels; stimulates the production of red blood cells to increase blood oxygen levels
3. pertaining to or containing nitrogen, usually the end product of protein metabolism
4. abbreviation for potential hydrogen, pH is a scale representing the relative acidity or alkalinity or a substance in which 7.0 is neutral; numbers lower than 7.0 are acidic and numbers above 7.0 are basic
5. the relative density of a substance (e.g., urine)
6. the final product of protein metabolism in the body and the main nitrogenous component in the urine
7. a by-product of protein metabolism present in the blood and excreted by the kidneys
8. stone formation in the renal pelvis that fills the chamber and assumes the shape of the calyces

Case Studies

1. Kidney stones are painful because they can lodge in any area of the urinary system (kidney, ureter, or bladder) and cause an obstruction. Some stones have rough edges that abrade the mucous membrane of the system. This can cause pain and hematuria. Lithotripsy is a procedure in which the kidney stone is crushed using ultrasound. The remnants of the stone can then be passed through the system and eliminated by the voiding process.
2. Glomerulonephritis is an inflammation of the glomerulus of the kidney. Symptoms may include mild edema, proteinuria, hematuria, and oliguria to complete renal failure. It is sometimes seen in children after a streptococcal infection. Strep antibodies, produced in response to the infection, attack and injure the glomeruli. Treatment for streptococcal infections with antibiotics has greatly reduced the incidence of poststrep glomerulonephritis, however, it remains a risk even with prompt treatment of streptococcal infections.

Charting Exercise

8/30/99 4:30 p.m.
c/o Lt flank pain x 3 hrs. Urine specimen obtained and urinalysis performed. IV pyelogram confirms calculi. Lithotripsy scheduled for tomorrow.

J. Williams, MA

Basic Writing Activities

Skill Drills

1. urea
   uric acid
   creatinine
2. 2 kidneys—remove the products of cellular metabolism from the bloodstream and aid in homeostasis
   2 ureters—transport urine from the kidneys to the bladder
   1 bladder—holds the urine until micturition (voiding or urination)
   1 urethra—tube that transports urine from the bladder to the outside of the body
3. An intravenous pyelogram is an x-ray examination of the kidneys and urinary tract requiring the injection of a radiopaque dye into the circulatory system. The dye is filtered by the kidneys to enhance visualization of the renal structures. A retrograde pyelogram is similar to the IVP except that the dye is not injected intravenously but is introduced through a catheter inserted into the ureters through a cystoscope.

Completion

1. erythropoietin
2. parathyroid hormone
3. one million
4. 160–180 liters (about 45 gallons)
5. 8 inches
6. 1½ inches
7. urinalysis

Innovative Activities

Labeling

Refer to Figure 19-3, Simplified Diagram of a Nephron.

CHAPTER 20

Vocabulary

Matching

1. d 3. e 5. a 7. c
2. g 4. f 6. b

Fill-in-the-Boxes

1. flagellum
2. spermatogenesis
3. prostate
4. penis
5. Cowper's glands
6. cryptorchidism

Case Studies

1. PSA or prostate-specific antigen is the name of a blood test used to determine levels of prostate-specific antigen in the blood. Elevated levels are present in men with prostatic cancer. The medical assistant should tell Mr. Adams that PSA is often used in conjunction with a DRE to evaluate the prostrate gland. It is also used as a screening test and is often used by health departments as a public service.
2. Acyclovir is not a cure for herpes genitalis. It is used as a palliative measure to reduce the severity of the symptoms.

Charting Exercise

11/11/99 10:30 a.m.

Urethral culture obtained by Dr. Smith and routed to lab. Rx for Acyclovir given to patient. Return appointment scheduled. Discussion with patient regarding use of acyclovir.

G. Skochko, MA

Basic Writing Activities

Skill Drills

1. the male distribution of hair
   deeper voice
   larger and heavier bone structure
   greater muscle mass
   generally higher production of red blood cells
2. chlamydia
   gonorrhea
   syphilis
   herpes genitalis
3. spermatozoa—1% to 5% of semen
   prostate secretions—60% of semen
   seminal vesicle secretions—30% of semen
   bulbourethral glands secretions—5% of semen
4. semen disorders
   systemic disease
   sexually transmitted diseases
   testicular disorders
   sexual dysfunction

Fill-in-the-Blanks

1. ductus deferens
2. 70–75 days
3. digital rectal exam, PSA
4. hydrocele
5. undescended
6. primary

Innovative Activities

Labeling

Refer to Figure 20-2, Diagram of a Human Spermatozoon.

CHAPTER 21

Vocabulary

Word Scramble
1. hirsutism
2. anovulation
3. amenorrhea
4. gestation
5. lochia

Matching

1. c	3. b	5. g	7. a
2. e	4. d	6. f	

Case Studies

1. Explain to Janet Williams that there is a formula for determining an expected date of delivery. The formula is called Nagele's rule, and reads "The first day of the last menstrual period (LMP) + 7 days – 3 months + 1 year." Mrs. Williams EDD is 12/26/99.

A simpler method involves adding 9 months and 7 days to the first day of the LMP, and the EDD is the same (12/26/99).

2. Explain to the new employee that TORCH is a complex of four fetal abnormalities risk factors, with the addition of "other."

T = toxoplasmosis (a protozoal infection spread by cat feces)
O = other
R = rubella
C = cytomegalovirus
H = herpes

Charting Exercise

5/11/99 10:00 a.m.
Pregnancy test positive. EDD 12/26/99.

N. Wilson, RMA

Basic Writing Activities

Fill-in-the-Blanks
1. menarche
2. 5 days
3. endometriosis
4. syphilis
5. hysterosalpingography
6. ovaries

Skill Drills
1. ectopic pregnancy—a gestation in which a fertilized ovum implants somewhere other than in the uterine cavity

   hyperemesis gravidarum—vomiting during pregnancy that becomes unrelenting and leads to dehydration, electrolyte imbalance, and weight loss

   abortion—termination of pregnancy or products of conception prior to fetal viability and/or 20 weeks gestation

   pregnancy-induced hypertension—hypertension directly related to the pregnancy

   placenta previa—placenta is implanted either partially or completely over the internal cervical os, making delivery of the fetus before the placenta difficult

   abruptio placentae—premature separation or detachment of the placenta from the uterus
2. Hormonal contraceptive methods
   - birth control pill—estrogen and progesterone or progesterone alone taken orally to prevent ovulation
   - birth control injection—injection of synthetic progesterone every 3 months to prevent ovulation
   - birth control implants—devices containing synthetic progesterone implanted under the skin to prevent ovulation

   Barrier contraceptive methods
   - male condom—sheath that fits over erect penis and prevents release of semen
   - female condom—sheath that fits in vagina, held in place with rings
   - diaphragm (with spermicide)—rubber cap that fits over cervix and prevents entrance of sperm
3. CST—usually performed in an outpatient facility or in a labor and delivery unit of the hospital. It is performed to determine how well the fetus will tolerate uterine contractions. Uterine contractions are induced, either by nipple stimulation or by administration of oxytocin to the patient; fetal heart tones and movements are monitored. Physician must be in attendance.

   NST—a noninvasive obstetric procedure used to evaluate the fetal heart tones and movement in relation to spontaneous uterine contractions. The NST may be safely performed in the medical office.
4. HRT benefits in menopausal women are: protects against cardiovascular and skeletal disorders and decreases the menopausal symptoms, such as hot flashes, depression, and drying of the vaginal mucosa.

Innovative Activities

1. 11/10/00
2. 02/27/00
3. 05/25/00
4. 07/04/00

CHAPTER 22

Vocabulary

Matching

1. a 3. a 5. a 7. e 9. d
2. b 4. c 6. c 8. c

Definitions

1. humidifier
2. congenital anomalies
3. aspiration
4. varicella zoster
5. well-child visit
6. neonatologist
7. autonomous
8. immunization

Case Studies

1. Remain with the child.
   Assist with the examination when appropriate.
   Hold the child during the preliminary work-up if possible.
   Have parent restrain or hold the child.
   Have parent remain within the child's sight.
2. The DPT (diphtheria, pertussis, tetanus) immunization may cause mild fever and soreness at the site of the injection. For fever and discomfort the parent may give acetaminophen preparation. For soreness at the site of the injection the parent may use cool compresses. If the child's fever is over 101° F and the child seems unusually irritable the parent should contact the pediatrician.

Charting Exercise

3/16/00 10:00 a.m.
DPT immunization given and instructions for care reviewed with mother.

J. Smith, MA

Basic Writing Activities

Skill Drills

1. Any five of the following:
   Never leave children unattended in the reception area or examining room.
   Toys should be examined frequently and replaced when damaged.
   Keep all medical equipment out of the child's reach.
   Place infant scales on sturdy table and never leave child alone on the scale.
   Store disinfection solutions away from patient area.
   Dispose of all sharps in proper containers.
   Practice stringent hand washing.
2. Obvious indicators
   Any one of the following:
   reports of physical or sexual abuse by the child
   previous reports of abuse in the family with current indicators
   conflicting stories about the incident or injury from the parents and the child
   injuries inconsistent with the history
   injury blamed on siblings or someone other than the parent
   repeated emergency room visits for injuries
   fractures, burns, or skeletal injuries of a suspicious nature
   Hidden indicators
   Any one of the following:
   dislocations
   nervous system trauma, particularly "shaken baby syndrome"
   internal injuries, particularly to the abdominal area
   Behavioral indicators
   Any one of the following:
   overly compliant, too eager to please
   passive avoidance, such as refusing to make eye contact, shrinking from contact
   extremely aggressive, demanding, rage-filled behavior
   role reversal, "parenting" the parent
   developmental delays (the child may be using energy needed for maturation to protect himself from abuse)
3. height
   weight

Short Answer Questions

1.
   a. oral
   b. oral
   c. rectal
   d. tympanic
2. apically
3.
   a. crying, resisting approach of medical staff, clinging to parent
   b. crying, resisting approach of medical staff, clinging to parent
   c. exploring environment, welcomes approach of medical staff, may leave parent to explore
4. any one of the following
   a. involve the parent; keep the parent in the child's view; approach the child slowly; use a soft, soothing voice; verbalize reassurance
   b. all of the above, plus: explain procedures in terms the child can understand; expect resistance; use a firm, direct approach; ignore negative behavior; restrain to maintain the child's safety; allow the child to hold a "security object"
   c. all of the above, plus: encourage the child to verbalize feelings; explain why the procedure is being done; have the child help as much as possible
   d. involve the child in decision making; involve the child in care; encourage and support questions
   e. discuss procedures in terms an adolescent can understand; be aware that adolescent may resist authority figures; be sure patient education includes information regarding smoking, alcohol, and in some cases, birth control and STDs

Innovative Activities

Refer to Figure 22-5, Pediatric Growth Charts.
Student to plot the following data:
Female child, 36 months old, 30 pounds, 35 inches tall
Female child, 10 months old, 16 pounds, 23 inches tall, head circumference 44 cm

CHAPTER 23

Vocabulary

Matching

1. d 3. a 5. b 7. c
2. e 4. f 6. g

Definitions

1. a sudden fall in blood pressure or cerebral hypoxia resulting in loss of consciousness
2. tan or brown macule found on elderly skin after prolonged sun exposure; also known as liver spots
3. activities usually performed in the course of the day, i.e., bathing, dressing, feeding oneself
4. premalignant overgrowth or thickening of the upper layer of epithelium or horny layer of the skin
5. conversion of the molecules of a substance from one form to another as in medication within the body
6. inability or difficulty in swallowing
7. computerized radiography using radioactive substances to assess metabolic or physiological functions within the body rather than anatomical structures

Case Studies

1. Live with family
   Group homes
   Long-term care facilities
   Skilled nursing facilities
2. The medical assistant should tell Mr. Jones's daughter that the care of the Alzheimer's disease patient is difficult. The medical assistant should encourage the patient's daughter to take care of herself and tell her that home care agencies offer respite care for family members. She should offer her information about community resources.

Charting Exercise

9/16/99 4:30 p.m.
Patient's daughter given information on community agencies that support families of Alzheimer's disease.

J. Adams, MA

Basic Writing Activities

Skill Drills

1. Write out instructions in easy-to-understand terms; use large print if the patient is vision impaired.

   Have the patient repeat instructions to you for reinforcement.

   Before leaving the office have patient show how he or she will perform the procedure.

   Give the patient a large appointment calendar and list times and days for treatment and medications to be crossed off as completed.
2. Any five of the following:

   multiple chronic illness that stresses the family's physical, emotional, and financial resources

   senile dementia

   bladder or bowel incontinence

   age-related sleep disturbances that interfere with caretaker's rest

   dependence on the caretaker for activities of daily living

   deepening confusion and scattered attention span

   increasing anger, hostility, or isolation

   increase in alcoholism or requests for narcotics or sedatives

   marked loss of interest in matters of health

   secretive behavior

   sharp mood swings from deep depression to euphoria

   giving away favored things
3. levodopa (L-dopa)

   anticholinergics

   antihistamines with anticholinergic action

Fill-in-the-Blanks

1. Parkinson's disease
2. elder
3. 40
4. any two of the following: diet, exercise, or safety
5. vitamins, protein, fiber
6. sugar, salt, fat
7. poor hearing, slow response

CHAPTER 24

Vocabulary

Matching

1. b 3. f 5. d
2. e 4. a 6. c

Definitions

1. light-proof film holders
2. processed film containing a visible image
3. the process by which x-rays are produced
4. physician who interprets the radiographs
5. not permeable to the passage of x-rays

Case Studies

1. Explain to Mrs. Adams that although there are potential adverse effects, today's x-ray machines are sophisticated and technologically advanced and that safety procedures are adhered to. The safety procedures include (1) reducing exposure amounts as much as possible; (2) avoiding unnecessary examinations; (3) limiting the area of the body exposed; (4) shielding sensitive body parts from the radiation; (5) evaluating the potential pregnancy status of female patients before performing examinations.

2. The medical assistant can help to alleviate Mr. Hersch's anxiety by being sensitive to his feelings, and explaining what to expect using nontechnical terms (leave the technical explanations to the physician). Also instruct him to increase his fluids after the exam so that he does not become constipated; this simple direction can save the patient much postexamination distress.

Charting Exercise

1/16/00 9:00 a.m.

Appears anxious, asking many questions, indicates concern that there will be discomfort during the examination, states has had "abdominal pain for 2 months" and "worried that the test will reveal an ulcer," and wonders if he will "have to take medicine or have surgery." Listened to concerns, explained procedure in simple, nontechnical terms. Seems less anxious at this time. Instructed to increase fluids after the examination in order to prevent constipation. Physician informed.

Joyce Martin, RMA

Basic Writing Activities

Skill Drills

1. verifying the patient's identity and the examination to be performed
   preparing the patient
   preparing the room
   performing the procedure
   processing the images
   interpreting the images (performed by the physician); not performed by the MA but is part of the process. Inform the physician when x-rays are complete and ready to read.
   filing the images
2. reducing the exposure amounts as much as possible
   avoiding unnecessary examinations
   limiting the area of the body exposed
   shielding sensitive body parts from the radiation
   evaluating the potential pregnancy status of female patients before performing examinations

Fill-in-the-Blanks

1. dosimeter
2. balloon angioplasty
3. laser angioplasties
4. light

Innovative Activities

Labeling

Refer to Figure 24-4, Standard Positions for X-ray Examinations.

CHAPTER 25

Vocabulary

Fill-in-the-Boxes
1. anaphylaxis
2. ecchymosis
3. hematoma
4. seizure
5. septic
6. hypothermia

Matching

1. d	3. a	5. g	7. c
2. f	4. b	6. e	

Case Studies

1. Explain to Allison that hypothermia is an abnormally low body temperature, with rectal readings below 95° F. The rate of onset of hypothermia is variable. Very cold air and immersion in cold water can cause rapid drops in core temperature. Basic management of hypothermia include handling the patient gently, removing wet clothing, and covering the patient to prevent further cooling. Give warm oral fluids only if evidence of active rewarming is seen. The patient should be alert and able to swallow easily before taking fluids. They must be able to control shivering to achieve active rewarming. Avoid drinks that contain caffeine, which constrict peripheral blood vessels, and alcohol, which dilates them. Warm beverages with sugar, such as hot chocolate, can be given to begin replacement of fuel the body needs to restore normal heat production. No oral fluids should be given to patients with changing levels of consciousness.

Frostbite: Windy, subfreezing weather creates the greatest risk for frostbite. Frostbite occurs when small body parts with a high ratio of surface area to tissue mass (fingers, toes, ears, and the nose) are exposed to extreme cold. Larger areas of the extremities are vulnerable in more profound cooling. This cold exposure causes tissues to freeze and cells will eventually die. The type and duration of contact are the two most important factors in determining the extent of frostbite injury. The combination of wind and cold is a dangerous factor in freezing. Superficial frostbite appears as firm and waxy gray or yellow skin in an area that loses sensation after hurting or tingling. Prolonged exposure can lead to blistering and eventually deep frostbite, which most often afflicts hands and feet. No warning symptoms appear after the initial loss of feeling. Freezing progresses painlessly once the nerve endings are numb. Skin becomes inelastic and the entire area feels hard to the touch. Superficial frostbite can be managed by warming the affected part with another body surface, for example, placing an ungloved hand over a cold spot on the cheek. Management for more than superficial frostbite is rapid rewarming after any system-wide hypothermia has been corrected. Deep frostbite should only be managed in the hospital to prevent further damage. Frostbite victims should be assessed for signs of hypothermia as well. Clothing offers good protection against weather only if it is loose enough to avoid restricting circulation. Tight gloves, cuffs, boots, and straps add to the danger.

2. At the inservice, explain the following:

Types of Shock

Hypovolemic shock—caused by the loss of blood or other body fluids. If hypovolemic shock occurs due to blood loss it can also be call hemorrhagic shock. Dehydration caused by diarrhea, vomiting, or heavy sweating can also lead to hypovolemic shock.

Cardiogenic shock—the most extreme form of heart failure, occurring when the function of the left ventricle is so compromised that the heart can no longer adequately pump blood to body tissues.

Neurogenic shock—caused by a dysfunction of the nervous system (as seen in spinal cord injury). The diameter of the blood vessels in the body can no longer be controlled. This leads to a dilation of the blood vessels. Once the blood vessels are dilated, there is not enough blood in the circulation to fill the body's need, thus causing shock.

Anaphylactic shock—an acute generalized allergic reaction that occurs within minutes to hours after the body has been exposed to a foreign substance to which it is over sensitive.

Septic shock—caused by a generalized infection of the bloodstream in which the patient appears seriously ill. It may be associated with an infection such as pneumonia or meningitis, or it may occur without an apparent source of infection, especially in infants and children. History reveals that the patient may have become ill suddenly, or the illness may been developed over several days. Fever is present initially; however, hypothermia develops and is a clinical sign suggestive of sepsis.

Signs and symptoms of shock

1. restlessness or signs of fear
2. thirst
3. nausea
4. cold clammy skin
5. pale skin with cyanosis at the lips, earlobes, fingers, and toes
6. rapid and weak pulse
7. low blood pressure

Management of the patient in shock (general guidelines):

1. ensure an open airway and breathing
2. control bleeding
3. administer oxygen
4. immobilize for possible spinal injuries
5. splint fractures
6. prevent loss of body heat (use a blanket)
7. transport to the closest hospital as soon as possible

Charting Exercise

5/14/00 11:00 a.m.

In today for a physical examination before leaving for college in the northeast. Says hobby is mountain climbing; is making plans for a mountain climb in November. Information given regarding the effects of hypothermia and protection from frostbite.

Sandy Gilbert, RMA

Basic Writing Activities

Fill-in-the-Blanks

1. Rule of Nines
2. myocardial infarction
3. allergen
4. hyperthermia
5. respiratory (and) circulatory
6. avulsion

Skill Drills

1. heat cramps—need for cooling and rest

   heat exhaustion—management is the same as for heat cramps in the early stages, but if hint of decreased mental status or unstable vital signs demands closer attention, aggressive cooling measures must be used (as described for heat stroke, if rectal temperature is above 39° C).

   heat stroke—demands rapid cooling; move patient quickly to a cool area, remove clothing, and place cold water, ice, or wet sheets on the patient's body. Concentrate on the core surface areas where the ability to cool central blood is greatest: the scalp, neck, axillae, and groin. The patient should be given oxygen and placed on a cardiac monitor. Transport to the hospital with continued cooling enroute is required.
2. appropriate emergency rescue service telephone number (usually 911)

   location of the nearest hospital emergency department that provides 24-hour emergency care

   telephone number of the local or regional poison control center

   list of procedures or training on what to do in an emergency situation

   list of all personnel who are trained in CPR (this should include all office and medical staff)

   location and list of contents of the emergency medical kit

   a protocol of responsibilities for each health care worker in the office
3. Eliminate the source of the burn. Note: in the event of an electrical burn, protect yourself from the electrical source before attempting to rescue the patient.

   Assess the patient's airway, breathing, and circulation.

   Remove all jewelry and clothing necessary to evaluate the burn.

   Wrap the patient in a clean, dry sheet.

   Administer oxygen.

   Keep the patient warm.

   Treat the patient for shock.

   Transport the patient to the hospital.
4. hand or hands at throat

CHAPTER 26

Vocabulary

Matching

1. e 3. f 5. b 7. c
2. a 4. g 6. d

Definitions

1. measurements for size or volume, as in calibrations on a syringe or pipette
2. the rising or lowering of a liquid at the point of contact with a solid; used to pull blood into a capillary tube or small pipette
3. a spinning motion to exert force outward, heavier components of a solution are spun downward
4. a detailed record of all hazardous substances kept within a site
5. acceptable range as established for an age, a population, or a sex; variations usually indicate a disorder
6. a substance used to react in a certain manner in the presence of specific chemicals to obtain a diagnosis
7. small portion of anything used to evaluate the nature of the whole

Case Studies

1. Information needed on a lab request form:
patient data base
patient birth date and gender
date and time of collection
physician's name and address or identification number
checklist of the test/s to be performed
other: source of the specimen, list of medication the patient is taking that may alter certain test results, directions for reporting (e.g., STAT), and total volume of a 24-hour urine specimen

2. Explain to Ms. Cochran that a blood glucose test is one of the most common laboratory tests done and that a small amount of blood is drawn from her arm and sent to the lab for testing, to determine glucose levels in the blood.

Charting Exercise

8/4/00 8:45 a.m.
Blood for a CBC is drawn, and urine obtained for a UA. Specimens labeled with lab request forms completed and sent to Universal Labs.

Georgia Meyers, RMA

Basic Writing Activities

Skill Drills

1. urinalysis
   blood cell counts
   hemoglobin
   hematocrit
   blood glucose
   cholesterol levels
   pregnancy test
   quick screening test for diseases such a mononucleosis and strep throat
2. diagnosing a disease
   following the progress of a disease
   meeting legal requirements (e.g., drug testing, a marriage license)
   monitoring a patient's medication levels
   determining the levels of essential substances produced by the body
   identifying the cause of an infection
   determining a baseline
3. automated cell counter
   microscope
   chemistry analyzer
   centrifuge
   refrigerator or freezer
   glassware
4. physical hazards (fire, broken glass, liquid spills)
   chemical hazards (acids, alkalis, chemical fumes)
   biological hazards (diseases such as HIV, hepatitis and tuberculosis)

Fill-in-the-Blanks

1. anticoagulant
2. toxicology
3. bacteriology
4. histology
5. cytology

Innovative Activities

Students to obtain copies of MSDS sheets and share the information in class.

CHAPTER 27

Vocabulary

Matching

1. c 3. a 5. b 7. f
2. g 4. e 6. d

Definitions

1. bibulous
2. centesis
3. obligate
4. swab
5. virology
6. mordant
7. agar

Case Studies

1. A rapid strep test tests for the pathogen group A beta hemolytic streptococcus or *Streptococcus pyogenes*, which causes streptococcal pharyngitis, one of the most common presenting infections in the medical office. The results are read in a few minutes while the patient waits. The advantage is that treatment can begin at once. Mary Smith presented with the symptoms of streptococcal pharyngitis. The rapid strep test enabled the physician to determine whether group A beta hemolytic streptococcus is present and begin treatment if the test is positive.
2. Dysentery is caused by a single-celled protozoan, entamoeba. The parasitology laboratory would perform cultures to identify the entamoeba organism.

Charting Exercise

3/2/00 9:30 a.m.

c/o fever 102 (orally) x 2 days, headache and sore throat x 1 day. Rapid strep test performed. Results positive. Rx for amoxicillin 250mg, 1 tab. qid x 10 days.

B. Watson, RMA

Basic Writing Activities

Skill Drills

1. Place a drop of the specimen on a glass slide with sterile saline or 10% potassium hydroxide (KOH).

   Place a coverslip over the specimen to reduce evaporation.

   To further decrease evaporation, place petrolatum around the rim of the coverslip.

   Inspect the slide by microscope using the high-power objective with diminished light.

   Place a drop of the specimen in the center of the coverslip with the petrolatum around the edge.

   Place the depression in the slide over the coverslip with the specimen in the center.

   Lightly press the slide against the coverslip to seal the edges; this will hold the slide tightly to the coverslip so that the specimen on the coverslip hangs into the depression on the slide.

   Inspect the slide arrangement by microscope with the high-power objective and diminished light.
2. Certain bacteria (cocci and bacilli) are capable of retaining crystal violet dye through a process to decolorize the specimen. Others are not capable of retaining the crystal violet dye. Those bacteria that retain the purple color are gram-positive. Those that do not are gram-negative and must be counterstained to be seen under a microscope. The gram-negative bacteria will retain a pink or red color from the counterstain. The staining of microorganisms helps the physician narrow the field of possible pathogens and initiate treatment before a culture has been incubated.
3. nutrients

   moisture

   proper pH

   temperature

   darkness

   presence or absence of oxygen

Short Answer Questions

1.
   a. P
   b. F
   c. P
   d. F
   e. F
   f. F
2. 1
3. Gram staining
4. positive
5. oxygen
6. sheep's
7. broth

Innovative Activities

Design a label to be attached to every specimen collection that includes all pertinent data:

Date specimen collected
Time specimen collected
Patient's name
Physician's name
Location from which specimen collected
Name of person who collected specimen
Name

CHAPTER 28

Vocabulary

Matching

1. d 3. c 5. b 7. a
2. e 4. f 6. g

Word Scramble

1. ammonia
2. culture
3. flocculation
4. lyse
5. electrolyte

Case Studies

1. Normal specific gravity range is 1.003–1.035; Mr. Wheaterby's urine specific gravity is within normal range at 1.030. Considering Mr. Wheatherby's history, Dr. Davies has probably ordered a specific gravity to determine the status of congestive heart failure. You know that high specific gravities can occur with congestive heart failure.

2. Yes, collect a clean-catch urine specimen. Normal urine will not contain bacteria, if collected properly. Bacteria present in significant amounts (more than a trace) is considered an indication of a urinary tract infection.

Charting Exercise

07/05/00 7:45 a.m.
Urine specimen collected and tested for specific gravity using a refractometer—results 1.030.

Joanne Nells, CMA

Basic Writing Activities

Skill Drills

1. physical examination
   chemical examination
   microscopic examination
2. renal disorders
   certain neoplasms
   urinary tract infections
   trauma to the urinary tract
3. Any six of the following seven:
   renal disorders
   certain neoplasms
   urinary tract infections
   trauma to the urinary tract
   transfusion reactions
   chemical toxicity
   burns
4. diabetes mellitus
   shock
   cardiac arrest
   malnutrition
   preeclampsia
   blood transfusion reactions

Innovative Activities

See Table 28-1 in the text for possible causes listed next to the given color and clarity of urine.

CHAPTER 29

Vocabulary

Matching

1. c 3. b 5. f 7. e
2. d 4. g 6. a

Definitions

1. any substance that inhibits the growth of bacteria; used on skin before any procedure that breaks the integumentary barrier
2. a bluish discoloration of the skin due to the lack of oxygen
3. an accumulation of fluid within the tissues
4. rupture of erythrocytes with the release of hemoglobin into the plasma or serum causing the specimen to appear pink or red in color
5. the palm surface of the hand
6. a complex substance found in blood and tissues that aids the clotting process
7. the small vessel that joins a capillary to a vein

Case Studies

1. blood culture–blood glucose–CBC: this "order of draw" avoids contamination of nonadditive tubes by additive tubes as well as cross-contamination between different types of additive tubes.
2. Signs and symptoms of latex allergy include redness, rash, itching at the site of latex exposure or hives, wheezing, angioedema, and bronchospasm. Treatment includes eliminating or reducing exposure to latex and administration of epinephrine and bronchodilators.

Charting Exercise

11/20/99 10:45 a.m.
Blood culture, blood glucose, and CBC drawn in order. Specimens routed to lab.

J. Smith, MA

Basic Writing Activities

Skill Drills

1. needle, syringe, and tube(s) or evacuated tubes
   tourniquet
   sterile gauze pads
   bandages
   needle and adapter
   sharps container
   70% alcohol pad or alternate antiseptic
2. Capillary blood specimens:
   finger
   heel
   big toe
   Venous blood specimens:
   cephalic vein
   median cubital
   basilic vein
3. Apply pressure for 3–5 minutes.
   Check the puncture site for bleeding and apply bandage.
   Cleanse the venipuncture or skin puncture site with an alcohol pad starting in the center of puncture site and working outward in a circular motion. Allow the site to dry or dry the site with sterile gauze. Do not touch the area after cleansing.

Fill-in-the-Blanks

1. oxygen
2. gloves
3. bleach
4. write identifying information with a pencil
5. small amounts
6. up

Innovative Activities

Design a label to be placed on a patient's chart that denotes a latex allergy.
Label should be large and of bright color with "latex allergy" clearly printed.

CHAPTER 30

Vocabulary

Matching

1. g 3. e 5. a 7. f
2. c 4. d 6. b

Definitions

1. one quadrillionth of a liter
2. a salt of folic acid; it acts to help enzymes that build structures such as blood cells
3. a condition of having increased numbers of dissolved substances in the plasma
4. small, sharp, spring-loaded instrument for quick capillary puncture
5. a naturally occurring anticoagulant given to prevent clot formation
6. an anticoagulant prescribed for patients likely to form blood clots, such as valve replacement recipients; also call Coumarin (trade name) or warfarin
7. a device for counting blood cells

Case Studies

1. Dr. Jones will use the partial thromboplastin time (PTT) test to monitor Mr. Allen's heparin therapy. A PTT will indicate how long it takes blood to clot. Heparin therapy will prolong the PTT, so this test is used for monitoring and determining dosages.

2. Explain to Ms. Peters that anemia is detected with a hemoglobin measurement, which is a direct indicator of the body's ability to oxygenate itself. The normal hemoglobin range for women is 12 to 16 g/dL.

Charting Exercise

04/14/00 9:00 a.m.

Blood specimen obtained for a hemoglobin test, lab request completed, and specimen sent to the lab. General information regarding hemoglobin tests requested and given. Also requests patient education information regarding types of anemia, brochures given.

Holly Gavin, RMA

Basic Writing Activities

Skill Drills

1. white blood cell count and differential
   red blood cell count
   hemoglobin determination
   hematocrit determination
   mean cell volume (MCV)
   mean corpuscular hemoglobin (MCH) and mean corpuscular hemoglobin concentration (MCHC)
   platelet count
2. chemical toxicity
   nutritional deficiencies
   chronic or overwhelming infections
   certain malignancies
3. infections
   inflammatory conditions
   certain drugs
   injuries to tissues
   certain malignancies
4. neutrophils
   lymphocytes
   monocytes
   eosinophils
   basophils

Fill-in-the-Blanks

1. whole blood
2. thrombocytes
3. clot
4. monocytes or lymphocytes
5. thromboplastin

Innovative Activities

See Figure 30-1 for answers to this labeling activity.

CHAPTER 31

Vocabulary

Matching

1. c 3. e 5. b
2. d 4. f 6. a

Definitions

1. jointed or paired
2. rupture of erythrocytes with the release of hemoglobin into the plasma or serum causing the specimen to appear pink or red in color
3. relating to a definite result
4. an underlying layer; a substance acted upon, as by an enzyme or reagent

Case Studies

1. Types of donated blood
autologous donation—patient's own blood, donated weeks before surgery
directed donor donation—donated by friends and family, cannot be given to anyone else
volunteer donor units—through the American Red Cross, blood is tested for ABO group, Rh type, unexpected antibodies to RBC antigens, and infectious agents; donors must give their medical history to protect the safety of the blood supply.

2. Explain to Jason (aged 15) that mononucleosis is caused by the Epstein-Barr virus and that adults present with symptoms of fatigue, malaise, sore throat, and enlarged lymph nodes. Infectious mononucleosis is usually self limiting and most patients fully recover.

Charting Exercise

10/03/00 3:20 p.m.
Blood specimen obtained for mononucleosis testing, lab request completed and specimen sent to lab. Requested information regarding mononucleosis. Educated to the cause, signs, and symptoms of mononucleosis.

Katherine Long, RMA

Basic Writing Activities

Skill Drills

1. identify bacterial and viral infections
   diagnose chlamydia infection, syphilis, and Rocky Mountain spotted fever
   measure substances found in pregnant women
   measure drugs in the urine
   measure hormones found in serum
2. kits maintained at proper temperature
   reagent protected against contamination by serum or other solution
   kits tested periodically for continued reactivity of all reagents
   a check performed each time the reagent is used
3. rheumatoid factor/rheumatoid arthritis
   infectious mononucleosis
   c-reactive protein
   rapid plasma reagin test for syphilis
   pregnancy test
   group A streptococcus
4. agglutination
   enzyme immunoassays (EIA)
   chromatographic assays

Innovative Activities

Educational brochures vary from one office to another. Students should obtain an example and create one focused on expectant mothers and RhoGAM.

CHAPTER 32

Vocabulary

Matching

1. f 3. d 5. c 7. e
2. a 4. b 6. g

Definitions

1. increases the rate at which a chemical reaction takes place. Example: Amylase found in saliva catalyzes (speeds up) the rate at which starches are broken down
2. a method of testing a patient's sensitivity or response to a substance by introducing it into the body and watching its effects
3. pertaining to or containing nitrogen, usually the end product of protein metabolism
4. the process of ascertaining the amount of something
5. a preliminary procedure, such as a test or exam, to detect the more characteristic signs of a disorder

Case Studies

1. Explain to Wanda Nagle that the ideal cholesterol range is 140–200 mg/dL; that when low-density lipoprotein (LDL) values are above normal range, the risk of heart disease is greater; and that when there are higher levels of high-density lipoproteins (HDL), there is a correlation with decreased risk of heart disease.

2. Explain to Mr. Jeffers that the normal range for an FBS is 50–110 mg/dL. A patient brochure on diabetes mellitus is given as the patient requested.

Charting Exercise

11/06/00 9:00 a.m.

Blood obtained for a cholesterol test. On request was given ideal cholesterol range. Educated to difference between higher levels of LDL and HDL.

Will return next week to obtain cholesterol test results. Appointment given.

Norma Mendoza, CMA

Basic Writing Activities

Skill Drills

1. bilirubin—normal values, direct: 0.4 mg/dL; total: 1.0 mg/dL
   alkaline phosphatase—normal values: 30–115 IU/L
   alanine aminotransferase—normal values: 0–45 IU/L
   aspartate aminotransferase—normal values: 0–41 IU/L
   total protein—normal range: 6–8 g/dL
   albumin—normal range: 3.6–5.2 g/dL
2. sodium (Na)
   potassium (K)
   chloride (Cl)
   calcium (Ca)
   magnesium (Mg)
   phosphorus (P)
   bicarbonate (HCO_3)
3. fasting blood glucose (sugar) (FBS)—a blood test—can be obtained from the patient after a 12–14 hour fast (nothing by water is taken during the fast). The normal range for FBS is typically 50–110 mg/dL.

   random blood glucose—a good screening tool, but is not as diagnostically useful as a fasting test. A random glucose can be drawn anytime during the day and has a slightly broader range: 45–130 mg/dL.

   2-hour postprandial glucose—usually used for individuals already diagnosed with diabetes. The patient must eat a high carbohydrate meal after a 12-hour fast. Two hours after the meal, a blood sample is drawn and glucose is measured. Timing of the specimen collection is extremely important in this test results. "Good control" of diabetes has been defined as a 2-hr pp of less than 130 mg/dL.

   glucose tolerance test (GTT)—used for diagnosing diabetes and hypoglycemia. The patient is challenged with a large dose of glucose, then blood glucose levels are checked at intervals to see how the body is metabolizing the glucose. Briefly, the GTT is performed by administering an amount of glucose calculated by the patient's weight. Blood is obtained 1/2, 1, 2, and 3 hours after the glucose has been administered. Blood sampling must occur at the precise times indicated for valid diagnosis. There are also special dietary, exercise, and smoking considerations in the days and hours just prior to the GTT test, and, in addition, the patient should have been free of illnesses during the previous 2 weeks.

Fill-in-the-Blanks

1. albumin
2. myocardium
3. artery
4. amylase
5. 45 mg/dL

Innovative Activities

Patient education brochures vary from one medical office to another. Students should obtain an example then create their own titled "Risk Factors for Premature Atherosclerosis and Coronary Heart Disease."

Guidelines for Responding to Critical Thinking Exercises

CHAPTER 1 ASEPSIS AND INFECTION CONTROL

Critical Thinking

Influenza (an example from Table 1-1)

Influenza is a viral infection spread by direct contact with individuals who are ill with the disease; by touching articles that have been touched by an individual with the illness; and by airborne droplets that are spread by coughing.

- Preventing the spread of the disease may be accomplished by:
- Washing hands **frequently, especially** before and after eating and when touching anything that has come in contact with the individual who is ill.
- Thoroughly washing all items that have been contaminated by secretions from the individual who is ill in hot, soapy water.
- Instructing the individual who is ill with the disease to sneeze, cough, and/or expectorate into tissue.
- Instructing the individual who is ill to wash hands frequently, especially after contact with any secretions.
- Placing tissues in a paper bag and disposing of it properly; the individual who handles the bag should wash his or her hands afterward.
- Receiving an annual immunization for influenza may reduce or eliminate the spread of this disease.

Procedure, Type of Asepsis, and Justification

- Catheterization—surgical asepsis. Urinary tract is normally sterile and surgical asepsis will prevent the introduction of any microorganisms into the area.
- Rectal temperature—medical asepsis. This area of the body is not normally sterile and medical asepsis will prevent the introduction of any pathogenic microorganisms.
- Excision of cyst—surgical asepsis. Surgical asepsis should be used when entering any part of the body considered to be sterile; any surgical procedure should be performed using surgical asepsis.
- Injection—surgical asepsis. Surgical asepsis should be used when entering any part of the body considered to be sterile; injections introduce a needle into body tissues or circulatory system.

Patient education handouts or brochures should be factual, clear, and concise. There are many formats that may be used. In this critical thinking exercise, the selected disease should be well defined with methods of transmission identified and prevention measures listed.

CHAPTER 2 MEDICAL HISTORY AND PATIENT INTERVIEW

1. Five interview techniques:
   Reflecting: Repeating back what you have heard, using open ended statements.
   Paraphrasing: Restating or repeating what you have heard, using your own words or phrases.
   Asking for examples: Asking the patient to give an example of the situation being described if you are confused about some of the information received.
   Asking questions: Asking open-ended questions that require the patient to formulate, answer, and elaborate on the response. Open-ended questions usually begin with "what," "when," or "where."
   Summarizing: Briefly restating the information you have obtained, or summarizing, gives the patient another chance to clarify statements or correct misinformation and helps to organize complex information or events.
2. "Good morning, Mr. Alvarez. My name is Lisa and I'm Dr. Martin's medical assistant. I want to ask you a few questions that will help the doctor plan appropriate care for you. Please be assured that your responses will be kept strictly confidential."

CHAPTER 3 ANTHROPOMETRIC MEASUREMENTS AND VITAL SIGNS

Critical Thinking

1. Effect of activity on blood pressure:
   Exercise raises the pressure.
   Depression will lower it.
   To obtain an accurate blood pressure reading, the blood pressure should be taken with the patient at rest. It is best to have the patient rest quietly in the examination room for a few moments before taking the pressure.
2. Choose the correct size of cuff before beginning to measure blood pressure. The blood pressure may be inaccurate by as much as ± 30 mm Hg if the cuff size is incorrect. A cuff too small will produce a reading that is inaccurately elevated and a cuff too large will produce a reading that is inaccurately low.

CHAPTER 4 PHYSICAL EXAMINATION

Critical Thinking

1. Auscultation involves listening to the sounds of the body. Palpation involves touching the body with the fingers or hands. Generally palpation is performed before auscultation. For the abdominal examination auscultation is performed before palpation because doing palpation may alter normal bowel sounds.
2. Assist the physician by handing the instruments and supplies needed and directing the light appropriately.

CHAPTER 5 INSTRUMENTS AND EQUIPMENT

Critical Thinking

1. Steam under pressure in the autoclave can be raised to a temperature higher than that of boiling water and is therefore more effective than boiling water in its ability to destroy bacteria, spores, and viruses.
2. Sanitation of instruments removes organic matter and residue and reduces the microbial population of the instruments. This step along with disinfection before sterilization ensures that the instruments will be free of all surface matter before being placed in the autoclave.

CHAPTER 6 ASSISTING WITH MINOR OFFICE SURGERY

1. Precautions to take when you are to shave and prepare a skin site prior to a minor surgical procedure:
   Use a new razor.
   Use soapy lather or shaving cream.
   Shave in the direction the hair is growing.
   Rinse well with warm water.
   Pat dry with gauze squares.
   Apply antiseptic solution of the physician's choice using sterile gauze, sterile cotton balls, or antiseptic wipes.

2. Epinephrine is added to local anesthetics to slow absorption by the body and lengthen its effectiveness, and as a vasoconstrictor to help provide hemostasis when the physician anticipates a longer procedure.

CHAPTER 7 PHARMACOLOGY

Critical Thinking

1. Any two of the following:
   Provide written instruction.
   Review directions for taking medication.
   Identify resources for further information.
   Alert patient regarding any precautions while taking a particular medication.
2. Answer unique to drug chosen by student. Student should site page in PDR as reference.

CHAPTER 8 PREPARING AND ADMINISTERING MEDICATIONS

1. Several formulas are used for pediatric dosage calculation. The method considered to be the most accurate involves calculating dosage by body surface area (BSA) and requires a scale known as a nomogram. The nomogram chart estimates the BSA according to height and weight. BSA is expressed in square meters. After obtaining the BSA average, the following formula is used:

$$\frac{\text{BSA in m}^2 \times \text{Adult Dose}}{1.7} = \text{Child's Dose}$$

2. The parenteral medication route would be the route of choice if a patient is NPO or the drug cannot be absorbed in the gastrointestinal system.

CHAPTER 9 INTRODUCTION TO ANATOMY AND PHYSIOLOGY

Critical Thinking

1. Homeostasis is the means by which the body maintains a relatively constant internal environment. Homeostasis manages the constant fluctuations of the body functions by keeping the internal environment within relatively narrow boundaries. Feedback refers to the information that comes to the body's sensors from the internal or external environment. Feedback either stimulates or depresses the mechanisms that maintain homeostasis. Positive feedback is an increase in a body function in response to a stimulus. Positive feedback reinforces, rather than opposes, the change that is occurring. Clot formation in response to an injury is an example of positive feedback. Negative feedback works against change and is a stabilizing mechanism. An example of negative feedback is CO_2. As carbon dioxide levels in the blood increase, the respiratory rate increases to increase the rate that CO_2 is expired into the air.
2. Levels of organization of the body:
   Atoms: Smallest component of an element.
   Molecules: Groups of atoms of a particular type.
   Cells: Complex arrangement of chemicals designed to carry out specific activities.
   Tissue: Collection of similar cells acting together to perform a particular function.
   Organs: Collection of various tissues and cells working together to perform a specific function.
   System: Group of organs that work together to perform a specific function for the body.

CHAPTER 10 ASSISTING WITH DIAGNOSTIC AND THERAPEUTIC PROCEDURES ASSOCIATED WITH THE INTEGUMENTARY SYSTEM

1. The cause of keloids is unknown, but it occurs most frequently in young women, especially during pregnancy, and in African Americans. The most common sites are the neck and shoulders.
2. Decubitus ulcers are caused by prolonged pressure to an area of the body, usually over a bony prominence. The pressure impairs blood supply and nutrition to the area. The most common sites are over the sacrum and hips, but they may also be seen on the back of the head, ears, elbows, heels, and ankles. The risk of a decubitus developing can be reduced by frequently turning a bedridden patient to relieve pressure and keeping the bed linen clean and dry. Special mattresses, pads, and pillows are also useful in prevention.

CHAPTER 11 ASSISTING WITH DIAGNOSTIC AND THERAPEUTIC PROCEDURES ASSOCIATED WITH THE MUSCULOSKELETAL SYSTEM

Critical Thinking

1. Axillary crutch: May be wood or aluminum; extends from the axillae to the floor.
   Lofstrand or Canadian crutch: Usually aluminum; reaches just to the forearms with a cuff to maintain its position on the arm with hand grip to distribute weight.
   Canadian crutches work well for individuals who need to use crutches for a longer period of time and also are easier to use for those individuals who have poor coordination.
2. A herniated disk is caused by severe trauma, degenerative changes, or strenuous strains. Symptoms include severe back pain, numbness in the extremities, spasms, weakness, and limitation of movement.

CHAPTER 12 ASSISTING WITH DIAGNOSTIC AND THERAPEUTIC PROCEDURES ASSOCIATED WITH THE NEUROLOGIC SYSTEM

1. The goal of long-term care for patients with spinal cord injuries is to prevent complications, which can include skin ulcerations, hypostatic pneumonia, bladder infections, contractures, and depression.
2. The reflex arc is part of the body's internal communication. A reflex is the body's involuntary response to a given stimulus. Reflex arcs are tested during routine office visits in what is commonly called reflex testing. The most common example is the tapping of the knee with a reflex hammer. The reflex arc sequence of events are: (1) the skin of the knee is stimulated by the hammer tap to the knee; (2) the sensory neuron transmits the impulse along a dendrite to the cell body of the neuron; (3) the sensory axon carries the impulse to the spinal cord; (4) the message is received within the spinal cord by the central neuron and transmission begins to the motor neuron dendrite; (5) the message is received and processed by the cell body of the motor neuron and is passed on to its axon; (6) the motor neuron axon stimulates the muscles in the knee to contract, causing movement to occur before the brain has had time to interpret the message sent by the ascending spinal nerves that the blow or knee tap has occurred.

CHAPTER 13 ASSISTING WITH DIAGNOSTIC AND THERAPEUTIC PROCEDURES ASSOCIATED WITH THE SENSORY SYSTEM

Critical Thinking

1. Otitis media, an inflammation or infection of the middle ear, frequently results from an upper respiratory infection (URI). Pathogens responsible for pharyngitis, nasopharyngitis, and the common cold frequently travel through the warm, moist eustachian tube to the middle ear and cause infection. As the infection progresses, the eustachian tube swells and closes off so that fluid that builds up does not drain. As the fluid increases, pressure on the tympanic membrane causes severe pain. Children have very short, almost horizontal eu-

stachian tubes which cannot drain well, thus they are more prone to ear infections. For many children every cold seems to advance into an ear infection. Any child who has an upper respiratory infection and complains of an earache should be examined by a physician to determine whether otitis media is present. Otitis media is treated with a 10-day course of antibiotics.

2. Strabismus is a misalignment of eye movements caused by muscle incoordination. Exotropic strabismus is a misalignment of eye movements caused by lack of muscle coordination. The eyes turn out. Treatment may include patching of the good eye to force the affected eye muscles to strengthen. In some cases, surgery may be required to correct the deviant muscle.

CHAPTER 14 ASSISTING WITH DIAGNOSTIC AND THERAPEUTIC PROCEDURES ASSOCIATED WITH THE ENDOCRINE SYSTEM

1. In simple goiter there is no clinical syndrome because there is no hyposecretion or hypersecretion of the gland. The gland is essentially normal, capable of manufacturing a normal concentration of hormone if iodine is supplied in the diet. However, the gland may become so enlarged that it compresses the trachea and other structures located in the neck. Under these conditions, the goiter must be surgically removed. Generally, in the early stages of goiter development, supplemental iodine can reverse the glandular enlargement. The value of iodine used prophylactically against goiter is now generally accepted and recommended for all areas low in natural iodine. The most feasible method of administration has been the addition of sodium or potassium iodide to table salt.
2. The physical effects of epinephrine secretion are:
   Contraction of arterioles, which increase blood pressure.
   Conversion of glycogen stored in the liver to glucose, which is rushed to muscle tissue for energy.
   Increased heart rate, which results in more blood for emergency response.
   Increased cellular metabolism, which boosts energy output.
   Dilation of the bronchi, which supplies more oxygen for metabolism.
   Decreased intestinal movement and activity and contraction of the cardiac, pyloric, ileocecal, and anal sphincters.
   Increased numbers of blood components and lymphocytes.

CHAPTER 15 ASSISTING WITH DIAGNOSTIC AND THERAPEUTIC PROCEDURES ASSOCIATED WITH THE CARDIOVASCULAR SYSTEM

Critical Thinking

1. Pernicious anemia is a deficiency in hemoglobin caused by a deficiency in vitamin B_{12}. Treatment is regular injections of vitamin B_{12}.

	CVA	*MI*
2. Proper medical term	Cerebrovascular accident	Myocardial infarction
Area affected	Brain tissue	Heart muscle
Symptoms	Numbness or tingling in face, difficulty swallowing, coughing or choking, slurred speech, unilateral vision disturbances, dizziness	Chest pain that lasts longer than 20–30 min., not relieved by nitroglycerin; dyspnea, nausea, diaphoresis, weakness, vomiting, and abdominal cramps
Treatment	Rehabilitation	Bypass surgery

CHAPTER 16 ASSISTING WITH DIAGNOSTIC AND THERAPEUTIC PROCEDURES ASSOCIATED WITH THE IMMUNE SYSTEM

1. Passive acquired natural immunity is acquired from another source, such as transplacentally from mother to fetus or through breast milk to a nursing infant from a mother who has immune factors. Passive acquired artificial immunity is acquired through the injection of gamma globulins after presumed exposure. Gamma globulins are not vaccines. Gamma globulins do not stimulate immune mechanisms but provide immediate antibody protection. Passive acquired artificial immunity is always temporary, lasting a few weeks to a few months.
2. The spleen has several functions, such as:
   Destroying old red blood cells.
   Cleansing the blood by filtration and phagocytosis.
   Producing all types of blood cells before birth and lymphoclytes and monocytes in adulthood.
   Serving as a reservoir for blood, which can be returned to the bloodstream in case of hemorrhage or other emergency.

CHAPTER 17 ASSISTING WITH DIAGNOSTIC AND THERAPEUTIC PROCEDURES ASSOCIATED WITH THE RESPIRATORY SYSTEM

Critical Thinking

1. It is better to inhale through the nose rather than the mouth because the nose is a defense mechanism of the respiratory system. It helps reduce the inhalation of viruses, bacteria, and foreign matter that could cause infection or damage to the respiratory tract and body. Hairs or vibrissae at the entrance to the nose filter large dust particles from the air. The mucous membranes in the nose trap dust and other particles and also add moisture to the air inspired. The turbinates in the nose whirl air around to increase warming, humidifying and additionally filtering the air.
2. Several actions taken by patients with COPD can improve their quality of life, that is, they can help the patient maintain optimal health. They include:
   Patient education- -to understand the disease process and what measures the patient can take to help himself or herself.
   Receive current flu vaccine and pneumonia vaccine.
   Supervised exercise program—maximize the use of lung function.
   Proper use of medications—reduce strain on lungs and heart.
   Good nutrition and fluid intake—support body's defenses against infection and increase viscosity of lung secretions to aid in expectoration.
   Home oxygen therapy to increase oxygen intake.

CHAPTER 18 ASSISTING WITH DIAGNOSTIC AND THERAPEUTIC PROCEDURES ASSOCIATED WITH GASTROINTESTINAL DISORDERS

1. There are two phases of metabolism: anabolism and catabolism. As part of the anabolic or constructive phase, digested nutrients are converted into units that can be absorbed and used by the cells for growth, repair, and each cell's specific functions. As part of the catabolic or destructive phase, these chemical units are broken down to release the energy stored within compounds.
2. You may tell the new employee that testing stool for occult blood using a test pack or kit is convenient, quick, and easy, and readily acceptable to most patients. This method is used widely for screening purposes to identify disorders that cause GI bleeding: hemorrhoids, polyps, diverticula, ulcers, or cancers. Several pharmaceutical companies manufacture test packs or kits to detect fecal occult blood. SmithKline Diagnostics supplies three methods: Hemoccult I, a simple slide for a single, simple test; Hemoccult II, with three test areas for collection from separate sites from three separate stools if intermittent bleeding is suspected; and Hemoccult Tape, for quick testing during rectal examinations. These tests use the guaiac reagent to indicate the presence of blood. Developers are added to the combination of stool and guaiac to turn the test site an indicated color. Universal precautions must be followed because stools not only contain bacteria, but may also contain hidden or occult blood.

CHAPTER 19 ASSISTING WITH DIAGNOSTIC AND THERAPEUTIC PROCEDURES ASSOCIATED WITH THE URINARY SYSTEM

Critical Thinking

1. Cystitis is more common in women than in men because the urethra of females is shorter (1½ inches vs. 8 inches in the male). Bacteria, therefore, have a shorter distance to travel to reach the bladder, where their presence causes inflammation. Female patients should be instructed to wipe from front to back after voiding or defecation to avoid the introduction of bacteria into the urethra.
2. Peritoneal dialysis offers the patient freedom to move about and continue a more normal lifestyle than hemodialysis. During hemodialysis the patient must remain connected to the dialysis unit for a period of 3 to 4 hours three times a week. Patients who have had extensive abdominal surgery with disruption of the peritoneal membranes are not good candidates for peritoneal dialysis. Systemic inflammatory disease and immunosuppression are also contraindications for peritoneal dialysis.

CHAPTER 20 ASSISTING WITH DIAGNOSTIC AND THERAPEUTIC PROCEDURES ASSOCIATED WITH THE MALE REPRODUCTIVE SYSTEM

Critical Thinking

1. Abstinence for the male would allow for the formation of increased amounts of sperm so that when ejaculation occurs more sperm would be available for fertilization.
2. Vasectomy, the bilateral removal of a segment of the vas deferens, prevents the passage of sperm from the testes. It has no effect on the production of semen, which forms the majority of the ejaculate.

CHAPTER 21 ASSISTING WITH DIAGNOSTIC AND THERAPEUTIC PROCEDURES ASSOCIATED WITH THE FEMALE REPRODUCTIVE SYSTEM

1. A patient education handout or brochure should be factual, clear, and concise. In this case the subject is herpes genitalis. The handout should describe the characteristics, causative virus, means of transmission, precautions, and possible treatment. The format for the handout will vary.
2. The decision to practice contraception and the selection of the appropriate method involves many factors. The patient's religious, cultural, and personal beliefs as well as the health history, financial situation, and motivation are all important considerations for both physician and patient. To reinforce the physician's advice and instructions, the medical assistant must be knowledgeable about the various methods, including the indications, risk factors, cost, and effectiveness. In addition, certain methods of contraception require the patient to undergo an invasive procedure. The group discussion should include all of the influencing factors noted above.

   Possible scenarios where factors would influence decisions: patient has strong religious beliefs against contraceptives; patient wants to use contraception, but does not want anything that could affect her physiology; patient has been using spermicides, but wants to switch to a hormonal contraceptive, however, she cannot afford an expensive method.

CHAPTER 22 PEDIATRIC PATIENTS

Critical Thinking

1. Safety tips for parents regarding administering oral medication:
   Hold infants in a semi-reclining position, not lying.
   Place the medication in the mouth on either side of the tongue.
   Use a medication spoon, syringe, dropper, or medicine cup.
   Administer small amounts of medication, allowing the child time to swallow.
   Explain the procedure at the child's level of understanding.

2. Well-child visits are scheduled at regular intervals depending on the child's age. The goal is to maintain the child's optimum health, which is accomplished by a complete physical examination and evaluation of the child's neurological and psychosocial development. Sick-child visits are made on an as-needed basis. The goal of these visits is the diagnosis and treatment of the child's immediate illness or injury.

CHAPTER 23 GERIATRIC PATIENTS

Critical Thinking

1. Passive neglect occurs simply through ignorance on the part of the caregiver as to the physiological and psychological needs of the patient. Many times caregivers are ill or elderly themselves and unable to supply the needs of the patient. Active neglect is the deliberate action taken by the caregiver to deprive the patient of care or a safe environment, or to render the patient passive and easier to care for by any means such as overmedicating.
2. The medical assistant is legally obligated to report suspicions of elder abuse to the physician who will assess the situation and then make a report to authorities. The majority of states now require that all suspected cases be reported to the Social Services Department.

CHAPTER 24 DIAGNOSTIC IMAGING

1. Legal tips you can give to a new employee are:
   Be sure radiographic images are properly identified.
   Keep in mind that interventional procedures require a consent form, similar to those used for surgical procedures, to be signed by the patient.
   Remember that only physicians are legally permitted to make a diagnosis or interpret radiographic images.
   Know your state laws regarding licensing for x-ray procedures: many states now require the licensing of all personnel who perform x-ray procedures, which may exclude medical assistants from taking x-rays.
2. You can tell a patient that following a barium enema, fluids should be increased to help to prevent constipation.

CHAPTER 25 MEDICAL OFFICE EMERGENCY

1. Dr. Lee will examine the pupils by quickly shining a flashlight at each eye from an angle about 6 to 8 inches from the eye. The patient should not look directly into the light. Both pupils should quickly constrict. Dr. Lee will examine the pupils for several items: equal size, dilation, constriction, constriction that occurs rapidly, reaction to light that is equal in both pupils.
2. The co-worker is choking. You ask "are you choking?" If the co-worker can not speak or cough the obstruction is complete. The first action is to stand behind the person and wrap your arms around the waist; make a fist with your non-dominant hand, thumb side against the patient's abdomen at midline between navel and xiphoid; grasp the fist with your dominant hand and give quick upward abdominal thrusts; completely relax your arms between each thrust and make each thrust forceful enough to relieve the obstruction.

CHAPTER 26 INTRODUCTION TO THE CLINICAL LABORATORY

1. You will tell other staff that spills can be avoided by pouring carefully; pouring at eye level if possible or practical and never pouring close to the face; tightly capping all containers immediately after use.
2. The type of personal protective equipment needed to draw a CBC is gloves, to prevent coming into direct contact with blood.

CHAPTER 27 MICROBIOLOGY

Critical Thinking

1. Culture media plates must be stored in the refrigerator with the side containing the medium uppermost. The plates should be stored in the plastic wrapper to keep the media moist. Petri plates stored with the medium downward may form condensation on the lids that will drip onto the surface, making it too moist for an accurate culture. The medical assistant should check the expiration date and the condition of the medium surface be-

fore using plates. Plates that are past the expiration date or any medium that has dried or cracked should not be used.
2. Streptococcal pharyngitis infection is caused by group A beta hemolytic streptococcus. Symptoms include fever, sore throat, and headache. It is treated with antibiotics.

CHAPTER 28 URINALYSIS

1. Because substances such as proteins, creatinine, and electrolytes are variably excreted during a 24-hour period, a 24-hour collection is a better indicator of values than a random specimen.
2. You can explain to the patient that avoiding contamination during a CCMS urine specimen collection is vital to obtaining an accurate test. You instruct males to not touch the penis to the inside of the container, properly clean the glans, and collect the urine in the middle of the urine stream. You instruct females to not allow the labia to close over the meatus, not let the urine stream run onto the labia or perineum, not touch the inside of the sterile urine container, and collect the urine at midstream.

CHAPTER 29 PHLEBOTOMY

Critical Thinking

1. Display a cheerful, confident, and pleasant manner.
   Introduce yourself.
   Explain the procedure in simple terms.
   Communicate effectively with the patient.
2. Capillary blood collection
   In infants under 3 months: prewarmed heel
   In older infants: big toe
   Warming the area can enhance blood flow

CHAPTER 30 HEMATOLOGY

1. The main operating principle of automated blood cell counters is a portion of whole blood (anticoagulated with EDTA) is taken in and diluted; these dilutions are moved into counting chambers where they are drawn through tiny holes (apertures), and as the cells pass through the holes, either an electrical current, a light beam, or a laser beam is interrupted. The instrument registers the interruption as a cell. It can tell the size of the cell by the length of time the beam is interrupted.
2. Elevations in ESR values are not specific for any disorder, however, they do indicate the presence of either inflammation or any other condition that causes increased or altered proteins in the blood. Physicians use this as a guideline when monitoring the course of inflammation in rheumatoid arthritis. ESRs can also be elevated with infections, pregnancy, and malignancy.

CHAPTER 31 SEROLOGY AND IMMUNOHEMATOLOGY

1. Syphilis is a sexually transmitted disease caused by a spirochete bacteria, *Treponema pallidum*. Incidence of the disease declined after World War II, but it has been increasing in recent years. The highest incidence is seen in individuals between the ages of 20 and 24. It can be transmitted from mother to fetus, resulting in congenital syphilis causing notched teeth, nerve deafness, and other symptoms. Syphilis is treated with penicillin.
2. Measles occurs most commonly in childhood. Today there is widespread immunization for rubella. In children and adults with measles, the symptoms are mild, low-grade fever and a rash on the face, neck, and truck. For a fetus of less than three months, measles can cause death or birth defects such as bone abnormalities, mental retardation, cataracts, and cardiovascular defects.

CHAPTER 32 CLINICAL CHEMISTRY

1. The pancreas functions in both the endocrine and exocrine systems and produces many secretions. Amylase and lipase, two of its exocrine system products, are released as excretory enzymes into the intestines to aid in digestion. Insulin and glucagon are hormonal products of its endocrine function and are released in the bloodstream to regulate carbohydrate metabolism.
2. Creatinine is a breakdown product of creatine, which aids in delivery energy to cells. Creatine is a chemical compound that adds phosphorus to adenosine diphosphate (ADP) to make adenosine triphosphate (ATP), the energy currency of the body.

Appendix
Externship Assessment Record

This list is a working tool between the clinical instructor and the externship supervisor to determine the students' ability to perform. It is an evaluation tool of what was learned and the ability to perform it. If any of these procedures are not observed during the students' externship, the externship supervisor should write "not observed" in the column provided.

G = Good **F = Fair** **P = Poor**

Name ____

Procedure	Date	G	F	P	Initials	Comments
Administering Oral Medications						
Administering Sublingual or Buccal Medications						
Applying Transdermal Medications						
Applying Topical Medications						
Preparing an Injection						
Administering an Intradermal Injection						
Administering a Tine or Mantoux Test						
Administering a Subcutaneous Injection						
Administering an Intramuscular Injection						
Administering an Intramuscular Injection Using the Z-track Method						
Measuring a Patient for Axillary Crutches						
Teaching a Patient Crutch Gaits						
Transferring to and from a Wheelchair						
Assisting with a Lumbar Puncture						
Preparing a Diagnostic Set						
Measuring Distance Visual Acuity						

continued

Procedure	Date	G	F	P	Initials	Comments
Measuring Color Perception						
Instilling Eye Medications						
Irrigating the Eye						
Assisting with Corneal Lavage						
Removing a Foreign Object from the Eye						
Performing Audiometry						
Irrigating the Ear						
Instilling Ear Medication						
Instilling Nasal Medication						
Performing a 12-Lead Electrocardiogram						
Mounting the ECG Strip for Reading						
Applying a Holter Monitor						
Collecting a Specimen for a Throat Culture						
Collecting a Sputum Specimen						
Preparing the Patient for Colon Procedures						
Administering an Intramuscular Injection Using the Z-Track Method						
Applying Cold Treatments						
Applying a Warm or Cold Compress						
Using a Hot Water Bottle or Commercial Hot Pack						
Assisting with Therapeutic Soaks						
Assisting with Cast Application						
Applying a Triangular Arm Sling						
Collecting a Stool Specimen						

continued

Procedure	Date	G	F	P	Initials	Comments
Testing for Occult Blood						
Assisting with a Pelvic Examination with a Pap Smear						
Assisting with a Colposcopy with Cervical Biopsy						
Assisting with the Insertion of an Intrauterine Device						
Assisting with the Removal of an Intrauterine Device						
Assisting with the Insertion of Subdermal Hormonal Implants						
Performing Nitroprusside Reaction (Accutest) for Ketones						
Obtaining a Clean Catch Midstream (CCMS) Urine Specimen						
Obtaining a 24-Hour Urine Specimen						
Determining Color and Clarity of Urine						
Determining Specific Gravity of Urine Using a Urinometer						
Determining Specific Gravity of Urine Using a Refractometer						
Performing Chemical Reagent Strip Analysis						
Performing a Copper Reduction Test (Clinitest) for Glucose						
Performing an Acid Precipitation Test for Protein						
Performing a Diazo Tablet Test (Ictotest) for Bilirubin						

continued

Procedure	Date	G	F	P	Initials	Comments
Preparing a Urine Sediment						
Performing a Microscopic Examination of Urine						
Obtaining a Blood Specimen by Venipuncture						
Obtaining a Blood Specimen by Skin Puncture						
Performing a Manual White Blood Cell Count						
Making a Peripheral Blood Smear						
Staining a Peripheral Blood Smear						
Performing a White Blood Cell Differential						
Performing a Manual Red Blood Cell Count						
Performing a Hemoglobin Determination						
Performing a Manual Microhematocrit Determination						
Performing a Wintrobe Erythrocyte Sedimentation Rate						
Determining Bleeding Time						
Performing a Mononucleosis Test						
Performing an HCG Pregnancy Test						
Performing a Group A Rapid Strep Test						
Determining Blood Glucose Using the Glucometer						
Glucose Tolerance Testing (GTT)						
Performing a Hemoglobin Determination						

Self-Study Program Instructions

System Requirements

A PC compatible computer with an Intel 386 or better processor. Windows 3.1 or later.
4 Megabytes of RAM (minimum); but recommend 8 MB RAM on Windows 3.1; or 8 Megabytes of RAM (minimum); but recommend 12 MB RAM minimum on Windows 95; and 3 Megabytes of available hard disk space.

Installation

Installing the Clinical Medical Assisting Self-Study program

1. Start up Windows.
2. Insert the disk into the floppy drive. From the Program Manager's File Menu, choose the RUN command.
3. When the RUN dialog appears, type a:\setup (or b:\setup if you are using b: as your disk drive) in the command line box. Click OK or press the "ENTER" button.
4. The installation process will begin. A dialog proposing the directory **"clinicalmed"** on the drive containing Windows will appear. If the name and location are correct, click OK. If you want to change this information, type over the existing data, then click OK.
5. When the setup routine is complete, a new group called **"CLINICAL MEDICAL ASSISTING"** will appear on your desktop.
6. Start the self-study program by double clicking on its icon.

The Clinical Medical Assisting Self-Study Program

This self-study program contains approximately 350 questions that review the content covered in the Competency Workbook to Accompany Lippincott's Textbook for Clinical Medical Assisting.
This is not a timed test. Take your time; consider the questions and the possible answers carefully. The Main Menu screen allows you to select which unit you would like to review. To begin a unit test, choose Start Test for that unit. To continue a test that you have already begun, choose Resume test. To re-start the test and erase your results from a previous test, choose Restart test. To review the answers you have given and compare them to the correct answers, choose Answers.
When you choose Start test, Resume test, Restart test, or Answers, the test and the program's Toolbar will appear.

Clinical Medical Assisting Toolbar

The Toolbar contains a series of buttons that provide direct access to all test program functions. When you move the cursor over a button, an explanation of its function displays in the Status Bar immediately above the Toolbar.
To get help at any time during the test, choose the Program Help button. Program help reviews basic functions of the program.
Answer each question by clicking on the oval to the left of an answer selection or by selecting the appropriate letter on the keyboard (e.g. A, B, C, D, etc.). When an answer is selected, its oval will darken. If you change your mind about an answer, simply select that choice, by mouse or keyboard, again.
To register your answer selection and proceed to the next question, click on the Right Arrow button or press Return.
After taking the test and receiving your score, you may review your answers by clicking on the Answers button on the Main Menu screen.
If you are unsure about an answer to a particular question, the program allows you to mark it for later review. Flag the question by clicking on the Mark button. To review all marked questions for a test, click on the Table of Contents button, which is immediately to the right of the Mark button.
The Table of Contents window lists every question included on the test and summarizes whether it has been answered, left unanswered, or marked for later review. Click on an item in the Table of Contents window and the program will move to that question. Use the Arrow buttons to move to the first, previous, next, or last question.
At any time during the test or when you are finished taking the test, click on the Stop button. If you wish, you may return to the session at a later time without erasing your existing answers by clicking on the Resume Test button on the Main Menu.
After taking the test, view the correct answer for each test question by using the Answers button on the Main Menu. This will take you back to the test, but you will not be able to modify the answers you have given. Click on the Q/A button (to the right of the Stop button), and a window pop up explaining the correct answer to the question. The Q/A button will only appear when you are in the Answer section of the test). You may also with to use the Table of Contents button to show you which questions you would like to review.

To exit the Clinical Medical Assisting self-study program, press the Quit button on the Main Menu.